Advanced Statistics for Kinesiology and Exercise Science

Advanced Statistics for Kinesiology and Exercise Science is the first textbook to cover advanced statistical methods in the context of the study of human performance. Divided into three distinct sections, the book introduces and explores in depth both analysis of variance (ANOVA) and regressions analyses, including chapters on:

- preparing data for analysis;
- one-way, factorial, and repeated-measures ANOVA;
- analysis of covariance and multiple analyses of variance and covariance;
- diagnostic tests;
- regression models for quantitative and qualitative data;
- model selection and validation;
- logistic regression

Drawing clear lines between the use of IBM SPSS Statistics software and interpreting and analyzing results, and illustrated with sport and exercise science-specific sample data and results sections throughout, the book offers an unparalleled level of detail in explaining advanced statistical techniques to kinesiology students. *Advanced Statistics for Kinesiology and Exercise Science* is an essential text for any student studying advanced statistics or research methods as part of an undergraduate or postgraduate degree program in kinesiology, sport and exercise science, or health science.

Moh H. Malek, Ph.D., FACSM, FNSCA, CSCS,*D, is an Associate Professor (tenured) of Physical Therapy in the Department of Health Care Sciences at the Eugene Applebaum College of Pharmacy and Health Sciences at Wayne State University in Detroit, Michigan, USA.

Jared W. Coburn, Ph.D., FACSM, FNSCA, CSCS,*D, is a Professor (tenured) of Kinesiology in the Department of Kinesiology at California State University, Fullerton, California, USA.

William D. Marelich, Ph.D., is a Professor (tenured) of Psychology in the Department of Psychology at California State University, Fullerton, and a consulting statistician for Health Risk Reduction Projects, Integrative Substance Abuse Programs (ISAP), Department of Psychiatry and Biobehavioral Sciences, David Geffen School of Medicine at the University of California, Los Angeles, USA.

Advanced Statistics for Kinesiology and Exercise Science

A Practical Guide to ANOVA and Regression Analyses

Moh H. Malek, Jared W. Coburn and William D. Marelich

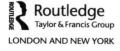

Routledge
Taylor & Francis Group

LONDON AND NEW YORK

First published 2019
by Routledge
2 Park Square, Milton Park, Abingdon, Oxon OX14 4RN

and by Routledge
711 Third Avenue, New York, NY 10017

Routledge is an imprint of the Taylor & Francis Group, an informa business

British Library Cataloguing-in-Publication Data
A catalogue record for this book is available from the British Library

Library of Congress Cataloging-in-Publication Data
Names: Malek, Moh H., author. | Coburn, Jared W., author. |
Marelich, William D., author.
Title: Advanced statistics for kinesiology and exercise science : a practical guide to ANOVA and regression analyses / Moh H. Malek, Jared W. Coburn, and William Marelich.
Description: Milton Park, Abingdon : New York, NY : Routledge, 2018. |
Includes index.
Identifiers: LCCN 2018010502| ISBN 9780415373012 (hbk) |
ISBN 9780415373395 (pbk) | ISBN 9781315231273 (ebk)
Subjects: LCSH: Kinesiology–Statistical methods.
Classification: LCC QP303 .M244 2018 | DDC 613.7072/7–dc23
LC record available at https://lccn.loc.gov/2018010502

ISBN: 978-0-415-37301-2 (hbk)
ISBN: 978-0-415-37339-5 (pbk)
ISBN: 978-1-315-23127-3 (ebk)

Typeset in Sabon
by Wearset Ltd, Boldon, Tyne and Wear

Books, especially those addressing quantitative methods, are not the sole product of their authors. We sincerely thank our families who have dealt with our moodiness as well as early morning and late-night writing sessions for this book. Without their support, only doodles would be within these pages. We also thank our students, where we've tested these concepts and appreciated their feedback. We would like to thank Jalen Weaver for his input on the cover.

Contents

PART III
Special statistical procedures   117

Figures

Tables

Part I
ANOVA analysis

1 What's stats got to do with it?

The word "statistics" can strike fear with many individuals whether they are undergraduate or graduate students, but also with many faculty members and researchers. This fear resides with the preconception that statistics are hard to perform. However, think about these questions, *"Do you know how to add and subtract numbers? Do you know how to multiply and divide numbers?"* If the answers to these questions are "yes," then you have a basic understanding of the foundation of statistics. With the advent of computers there came statistical software packages, therefore, you do not even have to add, subtract, multiply, and/or divide, because the program does those functions for you. What is important and most critical, however, is that researchers at all professional levels need to develop their skills to (1) understanding which statistical procedure(s) is appropriate to use for a given research question, (2) interpret the results, and (3) present the findings in a concise written manner.

In the context of our field, graduate programs related to kinesiology/exercise science may not require an extensive number of courses in statistics although this trend is starting to change. In addition, some departments outsource the statistical courses to another department such as psychology or public health. Herein lies the first challenge in learning statistics. That is, the kinesiology/exercise science student is not familiar with the terminology or assessment tools used in these other disciplines. As a result, the individual may have difficulty understanding which statistical procedure to use and how to interpret the output provided by the statistical program. Our goal here is to be discipline specific incorporating commonly used independent and dependent variables for each of the examples. For the faculty member a potentially different challenge is experienced. That is, they might rely on a biostatistician who may not always understand the nuances of the research question and/or measurement tools. Although we believe that biostatisticians are a beneficial part to the research team, it is imperative that the lead researcher has a strong knowledge and understanding of the statistical procedures they are using to answer their research question(s).

The overall goal of this textbook, therefore, is to expose the reader to the various advanced statistics techniques commonly seen in journals related to kinesiology/exercise science. Thus, we have refrained from presenting an exhaustive list of statistical procedures which are rarely used and/or require unique research designs that are outside the mainstream. Instead, we present a variety of statistical analyses which are commonly reported in journals related to kinesiology/exercise science. Moreover, detailed annotations of each statistical output from the IBM® SPSS® Statistics software (SPSS) statistical packages are provided to help facilitate the interpretation of the analyses. In addition, we also provide a sample write-up of the results which can be modeled when writing a thesis, dissertation, or manuscript.

There are, however, a few caveats to consider with this textbook. First, this was written with the assumption that the reader has completed an introductory statistics course covering basic conceptions and principles related to inferential statistics. At some Universities the introductory course may have been called *Measurement and Evaluation*, whereas other institutions refer to the course as *Introduction to Statistics*. Nevertheless, we will be building on this foundation of basic knowledge to provide the reader with more advanced skills. Second, we have primarily used SPSS to demonstrate the various statistical procedures, because of the ease with using the pulldown menus. However, we are aware that some of the more complex statistical procedures require syntax that cannot be derived from the pulldown menus. In such cases, we have provided the syntax which the reader will need to incorporate. Moreover, newer versions of SPSS may present their pulldown menu options differently than older versions. In such cases, we will provide instructions as needed. Lastly, we acknowledge that other statistical programs such as SAS and R are used and, in some cases, may be preferred over SPSS.

This textbook is divided into three sections (analysis of variance [ANOVA], Regression, and MANOVA). This approach was taken because ANOVA and regression are two of the most popular statistical techniques used in kinesiology/exercise science. As a practical matter, we wanted the reader to have the information on these two areas of statistics in one book that may be used as a pocket reference time and time again. Alternatively, faculty may use this textbook to teach ANOVA and Regression within the same semester or during the shorter summer semester over two sessions. Lastly, we have also added a third section called special statistical procedures. In this initial edition, we are introducing multivariate analysis of variance (MANOVA) and hope to add other more complex statistical procedures in subsequent editions based on feedback from the readership.

2 Organizing the data

Introduction

Prior to starting the formal statistical analyses, it is important to organize the data file in a manner where the correct statistical analyses will be performed. For simplicity and ease of use we recommend generating the data set in Microsoft Excel. In addition, importing the Excel file into SPSS is convenient (i.e., drag-and-drop in SPSS) and will maintain the majority of the formatting initiated in the Excel file.

Arranging the data

Typically, each row in the Excel file will be a study participant, whereas each column will be a variable (Table 2.1). Row 1 is usually used as the label for each column, because this will allow SPSS to use the first row as the label. Therefore, reducing time to re-label the SPSS file. In addition, make sure to use '_' to separate phrases when naming each column in the Excel file. This is important, because SPSS will not recognize spaces and in fact will delete spaces. Therefore, in the example below for weight, SPSS would label the column "Weightkg" instead of "Weight_kg." The latter version is easier to read and identify on the SPPS output.

If calculations are to be performed, we recommend performing all calculations in the Excel file before importing it into SPSS. For example, we calculated relative $\dot{V}o_2$ max from body weight and the absolute $\dot{V}o_2$ in liters per minute. Although SPSS has the "compute" command to perform the same calculations, it will need to be performed repeatedly if errors are detected for the variables of interest. For example,

Table 2.1 Arrangement of variables in Excel

Subject	Age	Weight_kg	$Vo_2max\_liters\_per\_minute$	$Relative\_Vo_2max$
1	22.0	70.0	4.5	64.3
2	25.0	72.0	4.2	58.3
3	23.0	80.0	4.6	57.5
4	21.0	81.0	4.0	49.4
5	22.0	86.0	4.0	46.5
6	24.0	88.0	3.5	39.8
7	26.0	82.0	3.6	43.9
8	22.0	75.0	3.9	52.0
9	23.0	74.0	4.5	60.8
10	24.0	88.0	4.3	48.9

using Table 2.1, the investigator typed 7 for the weight of subject #1 instead of 70. The relative $\dot{V}o_2$ *max* value would then be 642.9. In Excel this can be changed from "7" to "70" and the relative $\dot{V}o_2$ *max* value updates automatically to 64.2, whereas in SPSS the investigator would have to re-run the compute command to update the relative $\dot{V}o_2$ *max* column, because it will not automatically update that cell.

Organizing the data for ANOVA design

When performing analysis of variance (ANOVA) statistical procedures the investigator has to be cognizant of how the data are arranged. Unfortunately, SPSS will still perform the statistical analyses and **will not** recognize that the data were arranged in the incorrect format. Therefore, if the investigator wanted to examine $\dot{V}o_2$ *max* of individuals in three age groups (young, middle-aged, and old) the data should be arranged in the Excel file as shown in Table 2.2.

There are two options to labeling the group variable. First the investigator can use a similar labeling approach as shown in Table 2.2, or use the second approach by coding each group. That is, each group would be assigned a value as shown in Table 2.3. Therefore, the young group is coded "0," whereas the two other groups are coded "1" and "2," respectively. We suggest numerically coding the groups

Table 2.2 Depiction of the group variable for ANOVA design

Subject	Group	Age	Weight_kg	Vo₂max_liters_per_minute	Relative_Vo₂max
1	young	22.0	70.0	4.5	64.3
2	young	25.0	72.0	4.2	58.3
3	young	23.0	80.0	4.6	57.5
4	middle-aged	21.0	81.0	4.0	49.4
5	middle-aged	22.0	86.0	4.0	46.5
6	middle-aged	24.0	88.0	3.5	39.8
7	middle-aged	26.0	82.0	3.6	43.9
8	old	22.0	75.0	3.9	52.0
9	old	23.0	74.0	4.5	60.8
10	old	24.0	88.0	4.3	48.9

Table 2.3 Depiction of the group variable coded for ANOVA design

Subject	Group	Group_Coded	Age	Weight_kg	Vo₂max_liters_per_minute	Relative_Vo₂max
1	young	0	22.0	70.0	4.5	64.3
2	young	0	25.0	72.0	4.2	58.3
3	young	0	23.0	80.0	4.6	57.5
4	middle-aged	1	21.0	81.0	4.0	49.4
5	middle-aged	1	22.0	86.0	4.0	46.5
6	middle-aged	1	24.0	88.0	3.5	39.8
7	middle-aged	1	26.0	82.0	3.6	43.9
8	old	2	22.0	75.0	3.9	52.0
9	old	2	23.0	74.0	4.5	60.8
10	old	2	24.0	88.0	4.3	48.9

because it allows for flexibility with SPSS as some statistical functions require a numerical value to compute the statistical procedure(s). After coding the groups, the investigator can assign a label for each code, in SPSS, so that the SPSS data file looks like Table 2.3. We refer the reader to the SPSS manual on labels for the step-by-step approach to achieving this task.

Organizing the data for repeated-measures ANOVA design

Suppose that the investigator needs to examine 1 RM (repetition maximum) strength of 10 subjects at several time points. For example, the investigator wants to determine if a supplement would help increase 1 RM after 2 and 24 hours of ingestion compared to the initial 1 RM. In this case the investigator would arrange the data as shown in Table 2.4. Keep in mind that if this Excel table is imported into SPSS, there will be an "@" presented in front of the "1 RM" as such "@1RM." Therefore, if the user wants to avoid the "@" in their SPSS column then start the column with a letter such as "RM_1."

If the investigator was examining several groups, they would add a "group" column such as that shown in Table 2.5 to examine the differences between groups at each time point.

Table 2.4 Depiction of arranging the data for repeated-measures ANOVA

Subject	IRM_kg_PRE	IRM_kg_2h	1RM_kg_24h
1	70.0	76.0	79.0
2	63.0	69.0	72.0
3	80.0	86.0	89.0
4	88.0	94.0	97.0
5	84.0	90.0	93.0
6	71.0	77.0	80.0
7	72.0	78.0	81.0
8	77.0	83.0	86.0
9	60.0	66.0	69.0
10	63.0	69.0	72.0

Table 2.5 Depiction of arranging the data for repeated-measures ANOVA with a group variable

Subject	Group	Group_Coded	IRM_kg_PRE	IRM_kg_2h	1RM_kg_24h
1	young	0	70.0	76.0	79.0
2	young	0	63.0	69.0	72.0
3	young	0	80.0	86.0	89.0
4	middle-aged	1	88.0	94.0	97.0
5	middle-aged	1	84.0	90.0	93.0
6	middle-aged	1	71.0	77.0	80.0
7	middle-aged	1	72.0	78.0	81.0
8	Old	2	77.0	83.0	86.0
9	Old	2	60.0	66.0	69.0
10	Old	2	63.0	69.0	72.0

Organizing the data for regression analysis

Setting up the data file for regression analysis is the same as for ANOVA (see Tables 2.1–2.5). The only caveat is that dummy variables are needed when there are three or more levels of categorical variable such as in our group example (i.e., young, middle-aged, and old). For example, ethnicity is a categorical variable that could have three or more options. We present an example of dummy coding in the regression section.

Rules of thumb for organizing your data

Whether performing ANOVA or regression analyses, there are several rules to keep in mind as the reader is setting up their data file in Excel:

1. Always label each column (see Tables 2.1–2.5).

    a. Make sure to use '_' to separate out phrases so that once the Excel file is imported into SPSS the column titles are consistent with the Excel file.

2. Assign one column per grouping variable. That is, if there are two grouping variables (gender and experimental condition) then there will need to be two columns, whereas if there are three grouping variables (gender, experimental condition, and mode of exercise) then there will need to be three columns. In addition, make sure to numerically code each group (see Table 2.3) to facilitate the statistical analysis when importing the data into SPSS.

    a. *Caveat: when performing ANOVA via the General Linear Model function the investigator can use the "Group" variable that has string characters, Table 2.2. The investigator will, however, need to code the group variable for regression analyses especially if there are three or more variables.*

3. Each dependent variable (i.e., outcome measure) should be in its own column as shown in Table 2.1.

4. If certain variables need to be calculated, do those in Excel using the "function" feature before importing the data into SPSS.

    a. **Note:** For columns with numeric values perform the following steps in Excel:

        i. Highlight all the appropriate cells.
        ii. Designate those cells as "Number" using the Number Format.
        iii. Assign the appropriate number of decimal places.
        iv. Then save the file.
        v. If these steps are not performed, then SPSS will default each cell with numbers to 15 decimal places when the Excel file is imported.

5. If there are data missing for a subject, then leave that cell in the Excel file empty. When the file is imported into SPSS it will remain empty.

    a. **Note:** In some textbooks it is suggested to use "99" as the value for missing data rather than leaving the cell empty. The potential problem with using "99" or any other value to designate as "missing data" is that the user then needs to indicate, in SPSS, that designation or SPSS will calculate the "99" as a true data point.

6. Always check the data entry to avoid typos.
7. Save the Excel data file and then create a second duplicate Excel file that will be imported into SPSS. For example, the reader can save the original Excel file as "DataSet_1.xls" and then re-save as "DataSet_1_SPSS.xls" as this second file will be the one imported into the statistical program. This way, if there are issues with importing the Excel file into SPSS, the chances of the original data file becoming compromised are eliminated.

Importing your data file into SPSS

There are a number of ways to import the Excel file into SPSS and, therefore, we would refer the reader to the SPSS manual which will describe step-by-step procedures to successfully accomplish this goal. One simple approach, however, is to open SPSS and once the empty data sheet appears, drag-and-drop the Excel file into that data sheet and then select the options presented in the dialogue box that will appear.

3   Review of one-way analysis of variance (ANOVA)

Introduction

In this chapter, we provide a brief overview of ANOVA, whereas in subsequent chapters we will discuss in-depth advanced ANOVA designs.

Research questions

The types of research questions one can answer with one-way ANOVA are related to examining mean differences among groups. That is, the investigator may be interested in comparing mean differences between groups for a dependent variable. For example, the investigator needs to determine if mean differences exist for leg strength between male basketball players at three different conferences. Alternatively, the investigator may be interested in determining if there are differences in maximal oxygen uptake between marathon runners, cyclists, sprinters, and adventure racers, and if so, which group has the highest value.

The investigator also uses one-way repeated-measures ANOVA to determine if a dependent variable changes over time for a set of individuals. For example, the investigator may be interested in determining if muscle strength changes over a 5-week period in men. In this case, each subject would be tested weekly (week 1 to week 5) for an experimental period. As a result, a measure of weekly strength would be obtained. The one-way repeated-measures ANOVA would then allow the investigator to determine if there are differences in strength for that time period (i.e., 5 weeks).

Review of ANOVA

Prior to performing the formal analysis (i.e., ANOVA) it is important to make sure that the assumptions have been met. Our expectation is that the reader has been taught and understands the assumption of ANOVA in an introductory statistics course. In addition, we anticipate that the reader has knowledge of potential remedies that one would take if one or more of those assumptions are violated.

Typically, ANOVA is used when there are three or more groups as it is statistically inaccurate to perform multiple independent samples *t*-tests in place of ANOVA. One rationale, though there are others as well, is that multiple *t*-tests increase the *familywise error rate* which is related to maintaining the probability of falsely rejecting the null hypothesis below the alpha level, usually set at 0.05. It is also **critical** for the reader to remember that they **should not** perform multiple paired *t*-tests in place of one-way repeated-measures ANOVA without any adjustment to the alpha level. Again the same inflation in *familywise error rates* will occur which will invalidate your results and, therefore your conclusions.

Using SPSS pulldown menu for one-way ANOVA using General Linear Model

1. Click **Analyze**, then move cursor to General Linear Model and then move cursor to Univariate and then left click.
2. Click **Group**, then move to Fixed Factor(s) box.
3. Click **Relative_Vo$_2$max**, then move to Dependent Variable box.
4. Click **Post Hoc**.

   a. Click **Group** in the Factor(s) box and move to Post Hoc Tests for box.
   b. Check the box for Tukey which is Tukey HSD (Honest Significant Difference).

      i. Do not select Tukey's-b.

   c. Then click **Continue**.

5. Click on **Options**.

   a. Click on Group in the Factor(s) and Factor Interactions box and move to Display Means for box.
   b. Check the box for Descriptive statistics.
   c. The click **Continue**.

6. Click **OK**.

Syntax for one-way ANOVA using General Linear Model

UNIANOVA Relative_Vo$_2$max BY Group
/METHOD=SSTYPE(3)
/INTERCEPT=INCLUDE
/POSTHOC=Group(TUKEY)
/EMMEANS=TABLES(Group)
/CRITERIA=ALPHA(.05)
/DESIGN=Group.

Interpreting the output

As shown in Table 3.1, IBM SPSS Statistics software (SPSS) will generate the Tests of Between-Subjects Effects table. The Group variable shows that there is a significant overall *F*-ratio (9.233; $p = 0.011$). If the overall *F*-ratio was not significant ($p > 0.05$) there would be no further analyses. The investigator would conclude that there were no significant mean differences between the three groups for the outcome variable.

Since there was a significant overall *F*-ratio, a post-hoc follow-up test needs to be conducted to identify which groups are significantly different from one another. Therefore, SPSS first provides the Estimated Marginal Means table (Table 3.2) which is the data the investigator will use to report mean and standard error values for each group. Thereafter, SPSS provides a multiple comparisons table (Table 3.3).

Table 3.1 Tests of between-subject effects, reprint courtesy of International Business Machines Corporation

Dependent Variable: Relative_Vo$_2$max

Source	Type III sum of squares	df	Mean square	F	Sig.
Corrected Model	406.530[a]	2	203.265	9.233	.011
Intercept	27518.092	1	27518.092	1250.008	.000
Group	406.530	2	203265	9.233	.011
Error	154.100	7	22.014		
Total	27742.569	10			
Corrected total	560.630	9			

Source: © International Business Machines Corporation.

Note
a R Squared = .725 (Adjusted R Squared = .647).

Table 3.2 Estimated marginal means, reprint courtesy of International Business Machines Corporation

Group
Dependent Variable: Relative_Vo$_2$max

Group	Mean	Std. error	95% confidence interval	
			Lower bound	Upper bound
middle-aged	44.892	2.346	39.345	50.440
old	53.891	2.709	47.486	60.297
young	60.040	2.709	53.634	66.445

Source: © International Business Machines Corporation.

Table 3.3 Multiple comparisons, reprint courtesy of International Business Machines Corporation

Dependent Variable: Relative_Vo$_2$max
Turkey HSD

(I) Group	(J) Group	Mean difference (I–J)	Std. error	Sig.	95% confidence interval	
					Lower bound	Upper bound
middle-aged	old	−9.00	3.584	.091	−18.55	1.55
	young	−15.15	3.584	.010	−25.70	−4.59
old	middle-aged	9.00	3.584	.091	−1.55	19.55
	young	−6.15	3.831	.305	−17.43	5.13
young	middle-aged	15.15*	3.584	.010	4.59	25.70
	old	6.15	3.831	.305	−5.13	17.43

Source: © International Business Machines Corporation.

Notes
Based on observed means.
The error term is Mean Squared(Error) = 22.014.
* The mean difference is significant at the .05 level.

As shown in Table 3.3, there is a significant mean difference between the middle-aged and young groups ($p = 0.010$), whereas there is no significant mean difference between any combination of the other groups (p-values ranging from 0.091 to 0.305).

Sample write-up template

The one-way ANOVA revealed a significant overall F-ratio [F(df_{group}, df_{error}) = F-ratio value, p < 0.05]. The follow-up post-hoc Tukey HSD analysis indicated that Group A (mean ± SEM) had significantly larger strength index than Groups B (mean ± SEM) and C (mean ± SEM). In addition, we found that there was a significant mean difference between Group B and C.

Sample write-up for example

The one-way ANOVA revealed a significant overall F-ratio [$F(2,7) = 9.233$, $p = 0.011$]. The follow-up post-hoc Tukey *HSD* analysis indicated that individuals in the middle-aged group (44.8 ± 2.3 ml/kg/min) had significantly lower relative Vo_2max values than the young group (60.0 ± 2.7 ml/kg/min). There were, however, no mean differences between the young and old (53.9 ± 2.7 ml/kg/min) groups or the middle-aged and old groups.

4 Two- and three-way factorial ANOVA

Introduction

In Chapter 3 we briefly discussed one-way ANOVA which focuses on a single independent variable. In this chapter we will extend this concept to two or more independent variables. The use of factorial ANOVA is perhaps one of the most common statistical procedures used to analyze data in kinesiology/exercise science. This is because we often want to examine the *interaction* between at least two variables for a specific dependent variable. Although there are different variations of factorial ANOVA the primary focus of this chapter will be on two-way and three-way factorial ANOVA. Higher order factorial ANOVA such as four- or five-way are generally not recommended as they require more subjects per condition and more complex analyses the results of which are difficult to interpret (1).

Research questions

The types of research questions answered with two-way factorial ANOVA are those which examine the interaction between training and supplementation, or gender and age, on a dependent variable. For example, the investigator may be interested in determining the effects of a single dose of caffeine and endurance training status on time to exhaustion (4). In such a study, there would be an experimental "group" independent variable indicating individuals receiving a caffeine supplement or those receiving a sugar pill (a placebo), and a "training status" independent variable with two levels (trained individuals or novice individuals). This design, therefore, would be a 2 [group: placebo or supplement] × 2 [training status: trained or novice] factorial ANOVA. The investigator might employ such a design if they believe that the effects of supplement use on time to exhaustion depends on whether individuals are trained or novices. That is, whether there is an interaction between group and training status.

Review of factorial ANOVA

Factorial ANOVA is simply an extension of one-way ANOVA with the addition of another independent variable or variables. The same analysis process is undertaken, with variance partitioned into systematic and error variation. Multiple effects are now considered, including **main effects** (similar to the effects we see for a one-way ANOVA), and **interaction** effects of the independent variables. These are then followed up with post-hoc tests for the main effects, and simple main effects tests or planned mean comparisons for the interaction terms.

The assumptions of factorial ANOVA are similar to those applied in one-way ANOVA, and are applied to the independent variables and interaction cells on the dependent variable. Although generally robust to assumption violations, factorial ANOVA results are susceptible to bias especially when group sizes are disparate with unequal variances.

Independence of observations. As in one-way ANOVA, observations should be independent of each other. This is assessed by knowing your data. For example, are individuals in the sample related to each other (e.g., husband/wife)? If the investigator retained a sample of runners for a study from a local running club, such a dependency is possible.

Equality of cell sizes. Group or levels of the independent variable should be the same or approximately equal, including the cells for the interaction terms. If cells are not equal, the default Type III sum of squares performs an unweighted means analysis of the data which will make appropriate adjustments to the cell mean values to avoid a *condition effect*. Condition effects are biased findings in the main effect results for factorial ANOVAs due to the group means being differentially weighted based on their cell sizes. Type III sum of squares is the default in SPSS.

Even though the Type III sum of squares protects against condition effects, unequal cell sizes will continue to pose problems in terms of the other assumptions noted below. In particular, unequal cell sizes can heavily influence group variances, thus affecting homogeneity of variance. Very dissimilar group sizes should be avoided.

Normality. Dependent variable values should be normally distributed within each level of the independent variables and also within each cell of the interaction terms. This is assessed using histograms, box-whisker plots, and normality plots for the independent variable levels and interactions, looking for deviations from a normal distribution. Skewness and kurtosis may also be assessed, standardizing these values by dividing by their standard errors, and evaluating the resulting z-score value at a $p < 0.001$ value. Violation of normality is easily taken care of through transformations on the dependent variable.

Homogeneity of variance. Variances within each level of the independent variables and within each of the interaction terms is also required. Evaluating cell variances using a 9:1 ratio or less rule – placing the largest group variance over the smallest, called an *Fmax* test will usually suffice to assess this assumption, although if group sizes are vastly different or have small cell sizes, even small variance ratios (3:1) can lead to an inflated Type I error rate. In such instances, consider a more stringent alpha level (e.g., $p < 0.01$ instead of $p < 0.05$). For more complex factorial designs, Box's M test is also offered in SPSS to make this evaluation in aggregate (evaluated at a $p < 0.001$ cutoff).

Terminology

As we have mentioned previously, each statistical procedure has its own terminology to describe various components of the process. For factorial ANOVA the term *factor* refers to the independent variable(s). Therefore, in the above example, "group" and "training status" are factors and since we have two factors then we have a two-way factorial ANOVA. If, however, we wanted to add gender as a factor, then we would have three factors and conduct a three-way factorial ANOVA. In our 2×2 example, each factor has two **levels**. It should be noted that in a two-way factorial ANOVA a factor can have more than two levels. For example, we could add another group (i.e., elite athletes) to the training status factor such that our analysis would be a 2×3 factorial ANOVA, but still recognizing that it is a two-way ANOVA.

As a method of visualizing the statistical design, it is often helpful to draw out the conditions as shown below for a particular dependent variable. The main effect, therefore, examines the marginal means for each factor as shown below. Thus, a significant main effect for training status would indicate that overall, the trained group took longer to reach exhaustion than the novice group (75 vs. 40 minutes) regardless of which group there were assigned. Alternatively, a main effect for group would indicate that overall, caffeine increased time to exhaustion more than the placebo (70 vs. 45 minutes) regardless of training status.

Typically, when performing a two-way factorial ANOVA, we are interested in both the **main effects** (similar to effects noted in a one-way ANOVA), but more importantly in attaining a significant ($p < 0.05$) **interaction**. This means that one factor influences the effects of the other factor at a particular level (in some circumstances, this may be described as a *moderated* effect). Usually, the hypotheses in factorial designs will reflect the expected effects of the interaction between the independent variables. Both main effects and interaction effects are provided in the ANOVA summary table in SPSS, and are evaluated for significance ($p < 0.05$).

When significant main effects are attained, they are followed with a priori tests (e.g., contrasts), or *multiple comparison procedures* (e.g., Tukey HSD test). These are typical approaches followed in one-way ANOVA designs when there are three or more levels of an independent variable to evaluate mean differences. If there are only two levels of an independent variable in a factorial design (e.g., control vs. experimental group), the resulting F-test for the main effect directly assesses the group difference. In such a case, the investigator would look at the table of mean values provided in the output display.

When a significant interaction is attained, a number of approaches may be adopted. One approach is called a *simple main effect* test, which evaluates the systematic variance of one independent variable holding constant each level of the other independent variable on the dependent variable. For more complex designs (i.e., 3×3 factorial ANOVA), after simple main effect tests are performed, direct mean contrasts are required to further evaluate mean differences. Such a test could be the familiar *Scheffé test* which provides mean comparisons while controlling for family-wise error (i.e.,

Table 4.1 Depiction of the 2×2 factorial ANOVA

		Training status		
		Trained	Novice	
Group	Placebo	60	30	$\mu = 45$
	Caffeine	90	50	$\mu = 70$
		$\mu = 75$	$\mu = 40$	

Source: © International Business Machines Corporation.

holding the Type I error rate at the typical $p < 0.05$ level), utilizing the MS_{error} term from the factorial ANOVA in the formula (3). Another approach is to perform direct contrasts of the interaction cells of interest (based on the research hypothesis), again making appropriate adjustments to control family-wise error. In this case, again a *Scheffé test* with formula edits to reflect the factorial design could be utilized, *an a priori t-test* with a stringent alpha level (say $p < 0.01$), or the investigator could conduct *planned contrasts.*

Three-way ANOVA

The three-way ANOVA extends the two-way ANOVA by adding another factor to help explain the dependent variable. In three-way ANOVAs, main effects are produced, as are two-way interactions, and three-way interactions. Follow-up tests are the same as those used for two-way ANOVA, including the use of simple main effects or planned comparisons for the interaction terms.

Examples of two-way and three-way ANOVAs

Complete examples of two-way and three-way ANOVAs are presented below with annotations. For the two-way ANOVA, you have a 3 (group: control, placebo, or supplement) × 3 (training: 5, 10, or 15 days) with the dependent variable being strength. In the three-way ANOVA, you are interested in examining the effects of gender on the dependent variable in addition to the two conditions. Therefore, you have a 3 (group: control, placebo, or supplement) × 3 (training: 5, 10, or 15 days) × 2 (gender: male or female) with the dependent variable still being strength. Along with programming syntax and output for the factorial ANOVAs in SPSS, we also provide simple main effects tests.

Using SPSS pulldown menu for two-way factorial ANOVA

1. Click **Analyze**, then move cursor to General Linear Model, and then move cursor to Univariate and then left click.
2. Click **Group**, then move to the Fixed Factor(s) box.
3. Click **Days_of_training**, then move to the Fixed Factor(s) box.
4. Click **Strength**, then move to the Dependent Variable box.
5. Click **Plots.**

    a. Select group from the Factors box and move to the Separate Lines box.
    b. Select days_of_training from the Factors box and move to the Horizontal Axis box.
    c. Click **Add.**
    d. Click **Continue.**

6. Click **Options** (*in newer versions of SPSS you will need to click the EM Means box*).

    a. Select group from the Factor(s) and Factor Interactions box and move to Display Means for box.

   b. Select days_of_training from the Factor(s) and Factor Interactions box and move to Display Means for box.

   c. Select group* days_of_training from the Factor(s) and Factor Interactions box and move to Display Means for box.

   d. Check the box for Compare main effects.

   e. Choose Bonferroni from the pulldown menu for Confidence interval adjustment.

   f. In the Display box, check the box for Descriptive statistics.

   g. Click **Continue.**

7. Click **Paste.**
8. You will see the entire syntax for this statistical procedure which looks like the syntax below.
9. Before performing the analysis, however, you need to add a line of syntax which will provide the follow-up test for the significant interaction.

   a. This syntax is: /EMMEANS=TABLES(group*days_of_training) Compare (group) adj(BONFERRONI).

      i. This will allow us to examine mean differences between each length of training across the three groups.

   b. /EMMEANS=TABLES(group*days_of_training) Compare(days_of_training) adj(BONFERRONI).

      i. This will allow us to examine mean differences between each group across the three lengths of training.

10. After typing the above /EMMEANS syntax, press the green ▶ button to perform the statistical analysis.

Syntax for SPSS two-way factorial ANOVA

UNIANOVA strength BY group days_of_training
/METHOD=SSTYPE(3)
/INTERCEPT=INCLUDE
/PLOT=PROFILE(days_of_training*group)
/EMMEANS=TABLES(group) COMPARE ADJ(BONFERRONI)
/EMMEANS=TABLES(days_of_training) COMPARE ADJ(BONFERRONI)
/EMMEANS=TABLES(group*days_of_training) Compare(group) adj(BONFERRONI)
/EMMEANS=TABLES(group*days_of_training) Compare(days_of_training) adj
(BONFERRONI)
/PRINT=DESCRIPTIVE
/CRITERIA=ALPHA(.05)
/DESIGN=group days_of_training group*days_of_training.

Interpreting the output (two-way factorial ANOVA)

As shown in Table 4.2, SPSS will first show the Between-Subjects Factors. In this example, we can see that for the group factor there are three levels (control, placebo, and supplement) and for the length of training factor there are also three levels (5, 10, and 15 days). SPSS also indicates the number of subjects per level shown under the "N" column.

Table 4.2 Tests of between-subject effects, reprint courtesy of International Business Machines Corporation

		Value label	N
Group	1.00	control	15
	2.00	placebo	15
	3.00	SUPP	15
Length of training	1.00	5 days	15
	2.00	10 days	15
	3.00	15 days	15

Source: © International Business Machines Corporation.

As shown in Table 4.3, the Tests of Between-Subjects Effects table is generated which will indicate whether or not there are significant main effects for the group and days of training variables and/or a significant group×days of training interaction. Thus, we find no main effect for group ($p = 0.233$), but a significant main effect for days of training ($p = 0.000$, as shown) and a significant group×days of training interaction ($p = 0.002$). Since we have a significant interaction, we want to perform follow-up testing to determine where the mean differences exist.

As shown in Table 4.4, SPSS generates the Estimated Marginal Means table for the group×days of training interaction. It is these means and standard error values that you will use when reporting the data.

As shown in Table 4.5, SPSS generates the Univariate Tests table which indicates whether or not there is a significant overall F-ratio for the three length of training groups. This table is similar to the one-way ANOVA table and, therefore, we can see that for 5 and 15 days there are significant overall F-ratios ($p = 0.037$ and 0.003). Therefore, now we can look at the pairwise comparisons table. (**Note:** The Univariate Tests table appears after the pairwise comparisons table in the SPSS output.)

As shown in Table 4.6, SPSS produces the Pairwise Comparisons table which is generated from the syntax /EMMEANS=TABLES(group*days_of_training) Compare

Table 4.3 Estimated marginal means, reprint courtesy of International Business Machines Corporation

Dependent Variable: Strength Index

Source	Type III sum of squares	df.	Mean square	F	Sig.
Corrected Model	2934.400[a]	8	366.800	5.777	.000
Intercept	57245.000	1	57245.000	901.654	.000
group	192.933	2	96.467	1.519	.233
days_of_training	1418.133	2	709.067	11.168	.000
group*days_of_training	1323.333	4	330.833	5.211	.002
Error	2285.600	36	63.489		
Total	62465.000	45			
Corrected Total	5220.000	44			

Source: © International Business Machines Corporation.

Note
a R Squared = .562 (Adjusted R Squared = .465).

Table 4.4 Univariate tests, reprint courtesy of International Business Machines Corporation

1. Group* Length of Training

Estimates

Dependent Variable: Strength Index

Group	Length of training	Mean	Std. error	95% confidence interval	
				Lower bound	Upper bound
control	5 days	34.000	3.563	26.773	41.227
	10 days	35.600	3.563	28.373	42.827
	15 days	37.000	3.563	29.773	44.227
placebo	5 days	30.800	3.563	23.573	38.027
	10 days	31.800	3.563	24.573	39.027
	15 days	37.000	3.563	29.773	44.227
SUPP	5 days	21.000	3.563	13.773	28.227
	10 days	40.800	3.563	33.573	48.027
	15 days	53.000	3.563	45.773	60.227

Source: © International Business Machines Corporation.

Table 4.5 Pairwise comparisons, reprint courtesy of International Business Machines Corporation

Dependent Variable: Strength Index

Length of training		Sum of squares	df.	Mean square	F	Sig.
5 days	Contrast	458.800	2	229.400	3.613	.037
	Error	2285.600	36	63.489		
10 days	Contrast	204.133	2	102.067	1.608	.214
	Error	2285.600	36	63.489		
15 days	Contrast	853.333	2	426.667	6.720	.003
	Error	2285.600	36	63.489		

Source: © International Business Machines Corporation.

Note
Each F tests the simple effects of Group within each level combination of the other effects shown. These tests are based on the linearly independent pairwise comparisons among the estimated marginal means.

(group) adj(BONFERRONI). Here, you are determining which groups are statistically different from one another for each length of training. As we can see, for 5 days of training, the mean values for the control versus the supplement groups are significantly different from each other ($p = 0.042$). Similarly, we find that for the 15 days of training, there are significant mean differences between the placebo and supplement groups. It should be noted, that the mean differences are calculated in two ways thus the reason why one value has the negative sign and the other value is positive.

As shown in Table 4.6, SPSS has produced another Univariate Tests table. This was generated from the /EMMEANS=TABLES(group*days_of_training) Compare(days_of_training) adj(BONFERRONI) syntax. As mentioned above for Table 4.5, this is a one-way ANOVA table which will indicate if there is a significant overall *F*-ratio for any of

Table 4.6 Univariate tests, reprint courtesy of International Business Machines Corporation

Pairwise Comparisons

Dependent Variable: Strength Index

Length of training	(I) group	(J) group	Mean difference (I-J)	Std. error	Sig.[b]	95% confidence interval for difference[b]	
						Lower bound	Upper bound
5 days	control	placebo	3.200	5.039	1.000	-9.454	15.854
		SUPP	13.000*	5.039	.042	.346	25.654
	placebo	control	-3.200	5.039	1.000	-15.854	9.454
		SUPP	9.800	5.039	.179	-2.854	22.454
	SUPP	control	-13.000*	5.039	.042	-25.654	-.346
		placebo	-9.800	5.039	.179	-22.454	2.854
10 days	control	placebo	3.800	5.039	1.000	-8.8854	16.454
		SUPP	-5.200	5.039	.927	-17.854	16.454
	placebo	control	-3.800	5.039	1.000	-16.454	8.854
		SUPP	-9.000	5.039	.248	-21.654	3.654
	SUPP	control	5.200	5.039	.927	-7.454	17.854
		placebo	9.000	5.039	.248	-3.654	21.654
15 days	control	placebo	.000	5.039	1.000	-12.654	12.654
		SUPP	-16.000*	5.039	.009	-28.654	-3.346
	placebo	control	.000	5.039	1.000	-12.654	12.654
		SUPP	-16.000*	5.039	.009	-28.654	-3.346
	SUPP	control	16.000*	5.039	.009	3.346	28.654
		placebo	16.000*	5.039	.009	3.346	28.654

Source: © International Business Machines Corporation.

Notes

Based on estimated marginal means.

* The mean difference is significant at the .05 level.

b Adjustment for multiple comparisons: Bonferroni.

the three groups. Here, we see that the supplement group has an overall *F*-ratio that is less than $p = 0.05$. Therefore, we can continue on to the Pairwise Comparisons table.

As shown in Table 4.8, the Pairwise Comparisons table now provides information to determine which length of training statistically differs from one another for each group. Since we had a significant overall *F*-ratio for the supplement group, we examine the comparisons between length of training for the supplement group only.

As shown in Figure 4.1, SPSS produces a plot of the data. This was generated from the /PLOT=PROFILE(days_of_training*group) syntax. This graphical representation of the data typically appears at the end of the output display.

Sample write-up two-way factorial

The 3×3 factorial ANOVA revealed a significant group×training interaction [$F(4,36) = 5.21$; $p = 0.002$] for strength. In addition, there were no main effects for group [$F(2,36) = 1.52$; $p = 0.23$], but a main effect for training [$F(2,36) = 11.17$; $p < 0.001$]. The main effect for training was not interpreted due to the significant interaction (2), because the data cannot be collapsed across either factor. The follow-up analyses indicated that for the 5 days of training condition the supplement group had significantly lower strength index than the control group. For the 15-day condition, however, the supplement group scored significantly higher than the control and placebo groups.

Using SPSS pulldown menu for three-way factorial ANOVA

1. Click **Analyze**, then move cursor to General Linear Model, and then move cursor to Univariate and then left click.
2. Click **Group**, then move to the Fixed Factor(s) box.
3. Click **Days_of_training**, then move to the Fixed Factor(s) box.
4. Click **Gender**, then move to the Fixed Factor(s) box.
5. Click **Strength**, then move to the Dependent Variable box.

Table 4.7 Pairwise comparisons, reprint courtesy of International Business Machines Corporation

Dependent Variable: Strength Index

Group		Sum of squares	df.	Mean square	F	Sig.
control	Contrast	22.533	2	11.267	.177	.838
	Error	2285.600	36	63.489		
placebo	Contrast	110.800	2	55.400	.873	.427
	Error	2285.600	36	63.489		
SUPP	Contrast	2608.133	2	1304.067	20.540	.000
	Error	2285.600	36	63.489		

Source: © International Business Machines Corporation.

Note
Each F tests the simple effects of Length of Training within each level combination of the other effects shown. These tests are based on the linearly independent pairwise comparisons among the estimated marginal means.

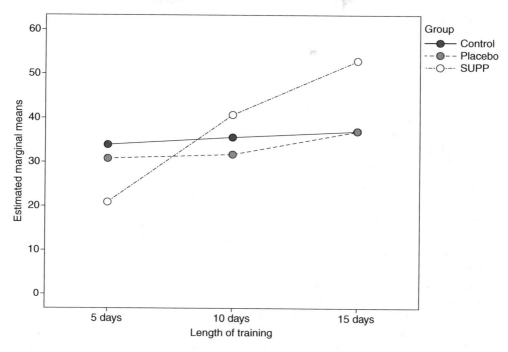

Figure 4.1 Estimated marginal means of strength index.

Source: © International Business Machines Corporation.

6. Click **Plots.**

   a. Select group from the Factors box and move to the Separate Lines box.
   b. Select days_of_training from the Factors box and move to the Horizontal Axis box.
   c. Select gender from the Factors box and move to the Separate Plots.
   d. Click **Add.**
   e. Click **Continue.**

7. Click **Options** (*in newer versions of SPSS you will need to click the EM Means box*).

   a. Select group from the Factor(s) and Factor Interactions box and then hold down the Shift key and then click group*days_of_training*gender variable.

      i. This will highlight all the variables and then you will be able to move them into the Display Means for box.

   b. Check the box for Compare main effects.
   c. Choose Bonferroni from the pulldown menu for Confidence interval adjustment.
   d. In the Display box, check the box for Descriptive statistics.
   e. Click **Continue.**

8. Click **Paste**.
9. You will see the entire syntax for this statistical procedure which looks like the syntax below.
10. Before performing the analysis, however, you need to add a line of syntax which will provide the follow-up test for the significant two-way interaction since, in this example, there will be no significant three-way interaction.

    a. /EMMEANS=TABLES(group*days_of_training)　Compare(group)　adj (BONFERRONI).

    b. /EMMEANS=TABLES(group*days_of_training) Compare(days_of_training) adj(BONFERRONI).

    c. After typing the above /EMMEANS syntax, press the green ▶ button to perform the statistical analysis.

Syntax for three-way factorial ANOVA

UNIANOVA strength BY group days_of_training gender
/METHOD=SSTYPE(3)
/INTERCEPT=INCLUDE
/PLOT=PROFILE(days_of_training*group group*gender)
/EMMEANS=TABLES(group) COMPARE ADJ(BONFERRONI)
/EMMEANS=TABLES(days_of_training) COMPARE ADJ(BONFERRONI)
/EMMEANS=TABLES(gender) COMPARE ADJ(BONFERRONI)
/EMMEANS=TABLES(group*days_of_training) Compare(group) adj(BONFERRONI)
/EMMEANS=TABLES(group*days_of_training)　Compare(days_of_training)　adj (BONFERRONI)
/PRINT=DESCRIPTIVE
/CRITERIA=ALPHA(.05)
/DESIGN=group days_of_training gender group*days_of_training group*gender days_ of_training*gender group*days_of_training*gender.

Interpreting the output (three-way factorial ANOVA)

As shown in Table 4.9, SPSS will first show the Between-Subjects Factors. In this example, we can see that gender is added as another factor in addition to the group and length of training factors. This additional factor (i.e., gender) changes the two-way factorial ANOVA into a three-way factorial ANOVA.

As shown in Table 4.10, the Tests of Between-Subjects Effects table is generated which will indicate whether or not there are significant main effects for group, days of training, and gender. In addition, there are the results of the two-way ANOVA and then the three-way ANOVA. First, examining the overall F-ratio for the three-way ANOVA (group×days of training×gender) indicates no statistical significance ($p = 0.914$). Since there is no significant three-way ANOVA, we now examine the two-way ANOVAs (days of training×gender; group×gender; and group×days of training). Here, the only interaction that is statistically significant is the group×days of training ($p = 0.003$). At this point, we want to perform the follow-up analyses for this interaction. We can report the main effects for group, days of training, and gender in our results section for completeness, but focus on the significant group×days of training.

Table 4.8 Between-subject factors, reprint courtesy of International Business Machines Corporation

Pairwise Comparisons
Dependent Variable: Strength Index

Group	(I) Length of training	(J) Length of training	Mean difference (I-J)	Std. error	Sig.[b]	95% confidence interval for difference[b]	
						Lower bound	Upper bound
control	5 days	10 days	-1.600	5.039	1.000	-14.254	11.054
		15 days	-3.200	5.039	1.000	-15.854	9.454
	10 days	5 days	1.700	5.039	1.000	-11.054	14.254
		15 days	-1.400	5.039	1.000	-14.054	11.254
	15 days	5 days	3.000	5.039	1.000	-9.654	15.654
		10 days	1.400	5.039	1.000	-11.254	14.054
placebo	5 days	10 days	-1.000	5.039	1.000	-13.654	11.654
		15 days	-6.200	5.039	.680	-18.854	6.454
	10 days	5 days	1.000	5.039	1.000	-11.654	13.654
		15 days	-5.200	5.039	.927	-17.854	7.454
	15 days	5 days	6.200	5.039	.680	-6.454	18.854
		10 days	5.200	5.039	.927	-7.454	17.854
SUPP	5 days	10 days	-19.800*	5.039	.001	-32.454	-7.146
		15 days	-32.000*	5.039	.000	-44.654	-19.346
	10 days	5 days	19.000*	5.039	.001	7.146	32.454
		15 days	-12.200	5.039	.062	-24.854	.454
	15 days	5 days	32.000*	5.039	.000	19.346	28.654
		10 days	12.200	5.039	.062	-.454	24.854

Source: © International Business Machines Corporation.

Notes
Based on estimated marginal means.
* The mean difference is significant at the .05 level.
b Adjustment for multiple comparisons: Bonferroni.

Table 4.9 Tests of between-subjects effects, reprint courtesy of International Business Machines Corporation

		Value label	N
Group	1.00	control	15
	2.00	placebo	15
	3.00	SUPP	15
Length of training	1.00	5 days	15
	2.00	10 days	15
	3.00	15 days	15
Gender	0.00	Male	22
	1.00	Female	23

Source: © International Business Machines Corporation.

As shown in Table 4.11, SPSS generated the Estimated Marginal Means table for the group × days of training interaction. It is these means and standard error values that you will use when reporting the data.

As shown in Table 4.12, SPSS generates the Univariate Tests table which indicates whether or not there is a significant overall F-ratio for the three length of training groups. This table is similar to the one-way ANOVA table and, therefore, we can see that for 5 and 15 days there are significant overall F-ratios ($p = 0.038$ and 0.005). Therefore, now we can look at the pairwise comparisons table. (**Note:** The Univariate Tests table appears after the Pairwise Comparisons table in the SPSS output.)

As shown in Table 4.13, SPSS produces the Pairwise Comparisons table which is generated from the /EMMEANS=TABLES(group*days_of_training) Compare(group)

Table 4.10 Estimated marginal means, reprint courtesy of International Business Machines Corporation

Tests of Between-Subjects Effects
Dependent Variable: Strength Index

Source	Type III sum of squares	df.	Mean square	F	Sig.
Corrected Model	3364.833[a]	17	197.931	2.881	.007
Intercept	55613.426	1	55613.426	809.395	.000
group	158.896	2	79.448	1.156	.330
days_of_training	1443.785	2	721.893	10.506	.000
Gender	149.833	1	140.833	2.050	.164
group*days_of_training	1419.926	4	354.981	5.166	.003
group*gender	155.400	2	77.700	1.131	.338
days_of_training*gender	68.422	2	34.211	.498	.613
group*days_of_training*gender	65.778	4	16.444	.239	.914
Error	1855.167	27	68.710		
Total	62465.000	45			
Corrected Total	5220.000	44			

Source: © International Business Machines Corporation.

Note
a R Squared = .645 (Adjusted R Squared = .421).

Table 4.11 Univariate tests, reprint courtesy of International Business Machines Corporation

Estimated Marginal Means
Group*Length of Training

Estimates
Dependent Variable: Strength Index

Group	Length of training	Mean	Std. error	95% confidence interval	
				Lower bound	Upper bound
control	5 days	33.667	3.783	25.904	41.430
	10 days	35.083	3.783	27.320	42.846
	15 days	37.333	3.783	29.570	45.096
placebo	5 days	31.833	3.783	24.070	39.596
	10 days	32.583	3.783	24.820	40.346
	15 days	37.083	3.783	29.320	44.846
SUPP	5 days	20.250	3.783	12.487	28.013
	10 days	41.333	3.783	33.570	49.096
	15 days	53.750	3.783	45.987	61.513

Source: © International Business Machines Corporation.

Table 4.12 Pairwise comparisons, reprint courtesy of International Business Machines Corporation

Univariate Tests
Dependent Variable: Strength Index

Length of training		Sum of squares	df.	Mean square	F	Sig.
5 days	Contrast	508.067	2	254.033	3.697	.038
	Error	1855.167	27	68.710		
10 days	Contrast	195.000	2	97.500	1.419	.259
	Error	1855.167	27	68.710		
15 days	Contrast	875.756	2	437.878	6.373	.005
	Error	1855.167	27	68.710		

Source: © International Business Machines Corporation.

Note
Each F tests the simple effects of Group within each level combination of the other effects shown. These tests are based on the linearly independent pairwise comparisons among the estimated marginal means.

adj(BONFERRONI). Here, you are determining which groups are statistically different from one another for each length of training. As we can see, for 5 days of training, the mean values for the control versus the supplement groups are NOT significantly different from each other ($p = 0.055$) as the p-value designated for statistical significance is $p \leq 0.05$. For the 15 days of training, there are significant mean differences between the control and supplement groups and the placebo as well as between the placebo and supplement groups. It should be noted, that the mean differences are calculated in two ways thus the reason why one value has the negative sign and the other value is positive.

Table 4.13 Univariate tests, reprint courtesy of International Business Machines Corporation

Pairwise Comparisons
Dependent Variable: Strength Index

Length of training	(I) group	(J) group	Mean difference (I–J)	Std. error	Sig.[b]	95% confidence interval for difference[b]	
						Lower bound	Upper bound
5 days	control	placebo	1.833	5.351	1.000	-11.824	15.491
		SUPP	13.417	5.351	.055	-.241	27.074
	placebo	control	-1.833	5.351	1.000	-15.491	11.824
		SUPP	11.583	5.351	.118	-2.074	25.241
	SUPP	control	-13.417	5.351	.055	-27.074	.241
		placebo	-11.583	5.351	.118	-25.241	2.074
10 days	control	placebo	2.500	5.351	1.000	-11.157	16.157
		SUPP	-6.250	5.351	.759	-19.907	7.407
	placebo	control	-2.500	5.351	1.000	-16.157	11.157
		SUPP	-8.750	5.351	.341	-22.407	4.907
	SUPP	control	6.25	5.351	.759	-7.407	19.907
		placebo	8.750	5.351	.341	-4.907	22.407
15 days	control	placebo	.250	5.351	1.000	-13.407	13.907
		SUPP	-16.417*	5.351	.015	-30.074	-2.759
	placebo	control	-.250	5.351	1.000	-13.907	13.407
		SUPP	-16.667*	5.351	.013	-30.324	-3.009
	SUPP	control	16.417*	5.351	.015	2.759	30.074
		placebo	16.667*	5.351	.013	3.009	30.324

Source: © International Business Machines Corporation.

Notes
Based on estimated marginal means.
* The mean difference is significant at the .05 level.
b Adjustment for multiple comparisons: Bonferroni.

As shown in Table 4.14, SPSS has produced another Univariate Tests table. This was generated from the /EMMEANS=TABLES(group*days_of_training) Compare(days_of_training) adj(BONFERRONI) syntax. As mentioned in the previous example, this table indicates whether or not there is a significant overall *F*-ratio for the three levels of group. In this example, the supplement group is the only one that has a significant overall *F*-ratio ($p = 0.000$; as shown). It should be noted, that when reporting *p*-values this small, a conventional method is to write $p < 0.001$.

As shown in Table 4.15, the Pairwise Comparison table now provides information to determine which length of training statistically differs from one another for each group. Since we have a significant overall *F*-ratio for the supplement group, we examine the comparisons between length of training for the supplement group only.

Sample write-up three-way factorial

The three-way factorial ANOVA revealed no significant group×training×gender interaction [$F(4,27) = 0.24$; $p = 0.91$] for strength. In addition, there were no significant ($p > 0.05$) gender×group or gender×training interactions. When the data were collapsed across gender, the two-way ANOVA revealed a significant group×training [$F(4,27) = 5.17$; $p = 0.003$]. It should be noted, however, that there were no significant main effects for group and gender, but a significant main effect for training [$F(2,27) = 10.51$; $p < 0.001$]. This main effect for training was not interpreted due to the significant interaction (2). The follow-up analyses indicate that for the 5 days of training condition the supplement group had significantly lower strength than the control and placebo groups, whereas this for the 15 days of training condition the supplement group had significantly higher ($p < 0.05$) strength than the two other groups.

Table 4.14 Pairwise comparisons, reprint courtesy of International Business Machines Corporation

Univariate Tests
Dependent Variable: Strength Index

Group		Sum of squares	df.	Mean square	F	Sig.
control	Contrast	32.822	2	16.4111	.239	.789
	Error	1855.167	27	68.710		
placebo	Contrast	77.400	2	38.700	.563	.576
	Error	1855.167	27	68.710		
SUPP	Contrast	2753.489	2	1376.744	20.037	.000
	Error	1855.167	27	68.710		

Source: © International Business Machines Corporation.

Note
Each F tests the simple effects of Length of Training within each level combination of the other effects shown. These tests are based on the linearly independent pairwise comparisons among the estimated marginal means.

Table 4.15 Pairwise comparisons, reprint courtesy of International Business Machines Corporation

Group	(I) Length of training	(J) Length of training	Mean difference (I–J)	Std. error	Sig.[b]	95% confidence interval for difference[b]	
						Lower bound	Upper bound
control	5 days	10 days	–1.417	5.351	1.000	–15.074	12.241
		15 days	–3.667	5.351	1.000	–17.324	9.991
	10 days	5 days	1.417	5.351	1.000	–12.241	15.074
		15 days	–2.250	5.351	1.000	–15.907	11.407
	15 days	5 days	3.667	5.351	1.000	–9.991	17.324
		10 days	2.250	5.351	1.000	–11.407	15.907
placebo	5 days	10 days	–.750	5.351	1.000	–14.407	12.907
		15 days	–5.250	5.351	1.000	–18.907	8.407
	10 days	5 days	.750	5.351	1.000	–12.907	14.407
		15 days	–4.500	5.351	1.000	–18.157	9.157
	15 days	5 days	5.250	5.351	1.000	–8.407	18.907
		10 days	4.500	5.351	1.000	–9.157	18.157
SUPP	5 days	10 days	–21.083*	5.351	.002	–34.741	–7.426
		15 days	–33.500*	5.351	.000	–47.157	–19.843
	10 days	5 days	21.083*	5.351	.002	7.426	34.741
		15 days	–12.417	5.351	.084	–26.074	1.241
	15 days	5 days	33.500*	5.351	.000	19.843	47.157
		10 days	12.417	5.351	.084	–1.241	26.075

Source: © International Business Machines Corporation.

Notes
Based on estimated marginal means.
* The mean difference is significant at the .05 level.
b Adjustment for multiple comparisons: Bonferroni.

References

1. Coburn JW, Housh DJ, Housh TJ, Malek MH, Beck TW, Cramer JT, Johnson GO, and Donlin PE. Effects of leucine and whey protein supplementation during eight weeks of uni-lateral resistance training. *Journal of Strength and Conditioning Research* 20: 284–291, 2006.
2. Keppel G and Wickens TD. *Design and analysis: a researcher's handbook.* Upper Saddle River, N.J.: Pearson Prentice Hall, 2004.
3. Kiess HO and Bloomquist DW. *Psychological research methods: a conceptual approach.* Boston: Allyn and Bacon, 1985.
4. Malek MH, Housh TJ, Coburn JW, Beck TW, Schmidt RJ, Housh DJ, and Johnson GO. Effects of eight weeks of caffeine supplementation and endurance training on aerobic fitness and body composition. *Journal of Strength and Conditioning Research* 20: 751–755, 2006.

5 Mixed or between-within factorial ANOVA

Introduction

Thus far we have discussed factorial ANOVA (one-, two-, or three-way) in which the dependent variable(s) was measured at a single time point. In Chapter 3 we briefly reviewed one-way repeated-measures ANOVA. Therefore, in the present chapter, we will combine components of both factorial and repeated-measures ANOVA which will allow us to examine different levels of one (or more) independent variable(s) in which each subject is measured on two (or more) occasions. This approach has different names, but typically it is called a *mixed factorial ANOVA*, or between-within ANOVA.

Research questions

In many kinesiology/exercise science studies, the goal is to examine the effect of a perturbation over several time points. For example, you may want to examine the effects of an 8-week endurance training intervention on time to fatigue. Therefore, you test all subjects (both control and experimental groups) before the intervention (pretest), at week 4, and at the end of the intervention (week 8). In this example you have a 2 [group: control or experimental] × 3 [time: pretest, week 4, and week 8] mixed factorial ANOVA in which the between-subjects factor is "group" and within-subjects factor is "time." Alternatively, you may want to examine the differences in electromyographic amplitude for the three superficial quadriceps femoris muscles (vastus lateralis VL, vastus medialis VM, and rectus femoris RF) in the same participants, but for two different modes of exercise. In this scenario, you would perform a 2 [mode: treadmill and cycle ergometry] × 3 [muscles: VL, VM, and RF] mixed factorial ANOVA in which the between-subjects factor is "mode" and the within-subjects factor is "muscles."

Review of mixed factorial ANOVA

The assumptions for a mixed factorial ANOVA are the same as for those of one-factor between-subjects ANOVA such as homogeneity of variance, normality, and independence of observation (for the between-subject independent variable). In addition, since we are also examining a within-subjects factor, we need to also examine compound symmetry which is assessed by the sphericity assumption when the repeated measures independent variables have three or more levels. The sphericity assumption is rooted in matrix algebra and essentially focuses on equal variance between a set of difference scores. The mathematical background related to discussing the sphericity assumption is beyond the objectives of this textbook, however, SPSS output provides the Mauchly's Sphericity test when performing repeated-measures ANOVA. The Mauchly's Sphericity test, therefore, is an indication of variance homogeneity. If this test is significant ($p < 0.05$) then we have violated the sphericity assumption, whereas a nonsignificant test indicates that the assumption has been met.

Mixed factorial ANOVA (example 1)

The example below focuses on the following research question *"Does treatment with a supplement increase running time to fatigue?"* Therefore, the research design is a 3 [group: control, placebo, and supplement] × 2 [time: pretest and post-test] with fatigue time as the dependent variable.

Using SPSS pulldown menu for mixed factorial ANOVA (example 1)

1. Click **Analyze,** then move the cursor to General Linear Model, and then move the cursor to Repeated Measures and left click.

   a. In the window that opens you will see the default "factor1."
   b. You can change this label or leave as the default "factor1."

      i. For our purposes, we will change this to "Time."
      ii. Then enter 2 for the number of levels, since we have two time points (Pre and Post).
      iii. Click **Add.**
      iv. Click **Define.**

2. Click **Group,** then move it over to the Between-Subjects Factor(s) box.
3. Click **Pre_Fatigue_Time.**

   a. Hold down the Shift key.
   b. Click on **Post_Fatigue_Time** (both Pre and Post variables should be highlighted).
   c. Move these two variables to the Within-Subjects Variables box.

4. Click **Plots.**

   a. Click **Group** and then move to Separate Lines box.
   b. Click **Time** and then move to Horizontal Axis box.
   c. Click **Add.**
   d. Click **Continue.**

5. Click **Post Hoc.**

   a. Click **Group,** and then move to the Post Hoc Tests for box.
   b. Click the box next to Tukey (do not click the box next to Tukey's-b).
   c. Click **Continue.**

6. Click **Options** (*in newer versions of SPSS, items "a–e" below are under the "EM Means" button*).

    a. Click **Group**.
    b. Hold down the Shift key.
    c. Click **Group*Time**.

        i.   You should have all 3 variables highlighted.
        ii. Move them to the Display means for box.

    d. Click the box Compare main effects.
    e. From the Confidence interval adjustment pulldown menu select Bonferroni.
    f. Click the box next to Descriptive statistics (*this is under "Options" in newer versions of SPSS*).
    g. Click **Continue**.

7. Click **Paste**.

    a. A syntax window will open (if one is not already opened).
    b. You will need to include the following /EMMEANS syntax, because they are not derived from the pulldown menu.

        i. /EMMEANS=TABLES(Group*Time) COMPARE(Group) ADJ (Bonferroni).

            1. This will allow us to examine mean differences between each group for each of the two time points.

        ii. /EMMEANS=TABLES(Group*Time) COMPARE(Time) ADJ(Bonferroni).

            1. This will allow us to examine mean differences between the two time points for each of the three groups.

        iii. The determination of which syntax line to use is dependent on the research question. It is, however, appropriate to have two separate research questions which would require using both syntax lines.

    c. After typing the above /EMMEANS syntax, press the green ▶ button to perform the statistical analysis.

Syntax for SPSS for example 1

GLM Fatigue_Time_pre Fatigue_Time_post BY Group
/WSFACTOR=Time 2 Polynomial
/METHOD=SSTYPE(3)
/POSTHOC=group(TUKEY)
/PLOT=PROFILE(Time*Group)
/EMMEANS=TABLES(Group) COMPARE ADJ(BONFERRONI)
/EMMEANS=TABLES(Time) COMPARE ADJ(BONFERRONI)
/EMMEANS=TABLES(Group*Time)
/EMMEANS=TABLES(Group*Time) COMPARE(Group) ADJ(Bonferroni)
/EMMEANS=TABLES(Group*Time) COMPARE(Time) ADJ(Bonferroni)
/PRINT=DESCRIPTIVE

/CRITERIA=ALPHA(.05)
/WSDESIGN=Time
/DESIGN=Group.

Interpreting the output for SPSS for example 1

As shown in Table 5.1, SPSS generates the Within-Subjects Factors table which are the two time points, whereas the Between-Subjects Factors table indicates the three groups. Therefore, all groups were tested at both time points.

As shown in Table 5.2, SPSS generates the Tests of Within-Subjects Effects table which provides information about whether or not there was a significant interaction and/or main effect for time. In this example, there was a significant group × time interaction ($p = 0.000$, as shown). In addition, there was a significant main effect for time ($p = 0.000$, as shown). However, because of the significant interaction, we only report the main effect for time, but do not conduct follow-up testing.

As shown in Table 5.3, the Tests of Between-Subjects Effects indicates that there is a main effect for group ($p = 0.030$). However, because of the significant interaction, we only report the main effect for group, but do not conduct follow-up testing.

As shown in Table 5.4, prior to the results of the pairwise comparisons SPSS provides the mean and standard error values for each group and time point. These are the values to use in when writing your results and/or generating graphs/tables.

As shown in Table 5.5, the Univariate Tests table is generated which indicates that there was a significant overall *F*-ratio for the second time point.

As shown in Table 5.6, the Pairwise Comparisons table shows that for the second time point, there are significant mean differences between the three groups. Keep in mind that this table was generated from the /EMMEANS=TABLES(Group*Time) COMPARE(Group) ADJ(Bonferroni) syntax line.

As shown in Table 5.7, another pairwise comparisons table is generated by SPSS from the /EMMEANS=TABLES(Group*Time) COMPARE(Time) ADJ(Bonferroni) syntax line. In this table, the comparisons are between the two time points for each group.

Table 5.1 Within-subjects factors, reprint courtesy of International Business Machines Corporation

Within-Subjects Factors
Measure: MEASURE_1

Time	Dependent variable
1	Fatigue_Time
2	Fatigue_Time_post

Between-Subjects Factors

		Value label	N
group	.00	control	10
	1.00	placebo	10
	2.00	SUPP	10

Source: © International Business Machines Corporation.

Table 5.2 Tests of within-subjects effects, reprint courtesy of International Business Machines Corporation

Tests of Withinw-Subjects Effects
Measure: MEASURE_1

Source		Type III sum of squares	df.	Mean square	F	Sig.
Time	Spherically Assumed	**110.677**	**1**	**110.667**	**103.745**	**.000**
	Greenhouse_Geisser	110.677	1.000	110.677	103.745	.000
	Huynh-Feldt	110.677	1.000	110.677	103.745	.000
	Lower-bound	110.677	1.000	110.677	103.745	.000
Time*group	Spherically Assumed	**72.742**	**2**	**36.371**	**34.093**	**.000**
	Greenhouse_Geisser	72.742	2.000	36.371	34.093	.000
	Huynh-Feldt	72.742	2.000	36.371	34.093	.000
	Lower-bound	72.742	2.000	36.371	34.093	.000
Error (Time)	Spherically Assumed	28.804	27	1.067		
	Greenhouse_Geisser	28.804	27.000	1.067		
	Huynh-Feldt	28.804	27.000	1.067		
	Lower-bound	28.804	27.000	1.067		

Source: © International Business Machines Corporation.

Table 5.3 Tests of between-subjects effects, reprint courtesy of International Business Machines Corporation

Tests of Between-Subjects Effects

Measure: MEASURE_1

Transformed Variable: Average

Source	Type III sum of squares	df.	Mean square	F	Sig.
Intercept	70402.246	1	70402.246	6387.545	.000
group	88.410	2	44.205	4.011	.030
Error	297.589	27	11.022		

Source: © International Business Machines Corporation.

Table 5.4 Group*Time, reprint courtesy of International Business Machines Corporation

Group*Time

Estimates

Dependent Variable: Strength Index

Group	Time	Mean	Std. error	95% confidence interval	
				Lower bound	Upper bound
control	1	33.170	.687	31.760	34.580
	2	34.275	.858	32.514	36.036
placebo	1	32.500	.687	31.090	33.910
	2	33.714	.858	31.953	35.475
SUPP	1	33.019	.687	31.609	34.429
	2	38.849	.858	37.088	40.610

Source: © International Business Machines Corporation.

Table 5.5 Univariate tests, reprint courtesy of International Business Machines Corporation

Univariate Tests

Measure: MEASURE_1

Time		Sum of squares	df.	Mean square	F	Sig.
1	Contrast	2.470	2	1.235	.262	.772
	Error	127.464	27	4.721		
2	Contrast	158.681	2	79.341	10.769	.000
	Error	198.929	27	7.368		

Source: © International Business Machines Corporation.

Note

Each F tests the simple effects of group within each level combination of the other effects shown. These tests are based on the linearly independent pairwise comparisons among the estimated marginal means.

Table 5.6 Pairwise comparisons, reprint courtesy of International Business Machines Corporation

Pairwise Comparisons

Measure: MEASURE_1

Time	(I) group	(J) group	Mean difference (I–J)	Std. error	Sig.[b]	95% confidence interval for difference[b]	
						Lower bound	Upper bound
1	control	placebo	.670	.972	1.000	-1.810	3.150
		SUPP	.151	.972	1.000	-2.329	2.631
	placebo	control	-.670	.972	1.000	-3.150	1.810
		SUPP	-.519	.972	1.000	-2.999	1.961
	SUPP	control	-.151	.972	1.000	-2.631	2.329
		placebo	.519	.972	1.000	-1.961	2.999
2	control	placebo	.561	1.214	1.000	-2.537	3.659
		SUPP	-4.574*	1.214	.002	-7.672	-1.476
	placebo	control	-.561	1.214	1.000	-3.659	2.537
		SUPP	-5.135*	1.214	.001	-3.659	2.537
	SUPP	control	4.574*	1.214	.002	1.476	7.672
		placebo	5.135*	1.214	.001	2.037	8.233

Source: © International Business Machines Corporation.

Notes

Based on estimated marginal means.

* The mean difference is significant at the .05 level.

b Adjustment for multiple comparisons: Bonferroni.

Table 5.7 Pairwise comparisons, reprint courtesy of International Business Machines Corporation

Pairwise Comparisons
Measure: MEASURE_1

Group	(I) time	(J) time	Mean difference (I–J)	Std. error	Sig.[b]	95% confidence interval for difference[b]	
						Lower bound	Upper bound
control	1	2	–1.105*	.462	.024	–2.053	–.157
	2	1	1.105*	.462	.024	.157	2.053
placebo	1	2	–1.214*	.462	.014	–2.162	–.266
	2	1	1.214*	.462	.014	.266	2.162
SUPP	1	2	–5.830*	.462	.000	–6.778	–4.882
	2	1	5.830*	.462	.000	4.882	6.778

Source: © International Business Machines Corporation.

Notes
Based on estimated marginal means.
* The mean difference is significant at the .05 level.
b Adjustment for multiple comparisons: Bonferroni.

Sample write-up for example 1

The 2×3 mixed factorial ANOVA revealed a significant group $\times$ time interaction [$F(2,27) = 34.09$; $p < 0.001$] for fatigue time. In addition, there were significant main effects for group [$F(2,27) = 4.01$; $p = 0.03$] and time [$F(1,27) = 103.75$; $p < 0.001$], however, these main effects were not interpreted given the significant interaction. The follow-up analyses indicate no significant mean differences between groups in the pretest fatigue time, but significant mean differences in post-test fatigue time. As a result, the supplement group had significantly higher post-test fatigue times compared to the control and placebo groups.

Mixed factorial ANOVA (example 2)

The example below focuses on the following research question "*Is there a mean difference in EMG amplitude in the thigh muscles between treadmill exercise and cycle ergometry?*" Therefore, the design is a 2 [mode: treadmill and cycle ergometry] $\times$ 3 [muscles: VL, VM, and RF] with EMG amplitude as the dependent variable.

Using SPSS pulldown menu for mixed factorial ANOVA (example 2)

1. Click **Analyze**, then move the cursor to General Linear Model, and then move the cursor to Repeated Measures and left click.

    a. In the window that opens you will see the default "factor1."
    b. You can change this label or leave as the default "factor1."

        i. For our purposes, we will change this to "EMG_Amplitude."
        ii. Then enter 3 for the number of levels, since we have three muscles (vastus lateralis, rectus femoris, and vastus medialis).
        iii. Click **Add**.
        iv. Click **Define**.

2. Click **Mode_of_Exercise**, then move it over to the Between-Subjects Factor(s) box.
3. Click **Peak_EMG_Amplitude_VL**.

    a. Hold down the Shift key.
    b. Click on **Peak_EMG_Amplitude_VM** (all three variables should be highlighted).
    c. Move these three variables to the Within-Subjects Variables box.

4. Click **Plots**.

    a. Click **Mode_of_Exercise** and then move to Separate Lines box.
    b. Click **EMG_Amplitude** and then move to Horizontal Axis box.
    c. Click **Add**.
    d. Click **Continue**.

5. Click **Options** (*in newer versions of SPSS, items "a–e" below are under the "EM Means" button*).

    a. Click Mode_of_Exercise.
    b. Hold down the Shift key.

    c.   Click Mode_of_Exercise*EMG_Amplitude.

        i.   You should have all three variables highlighted.

        ii.   Move them to the Display means for box.

    d.   Click the box Compare main effects.

    e.   From the Confidence interval adjustment pulldown menu select Bonferroni.

    f.   Click the box next to Descriptive statistics.

    g.   Click **Continue**.

6.   Click **Paste**.

    a.   A syntax window will open (if one is not already opened).

    b.   You will need to include the following /EMMEANS syntax, because they are not derived from the pulldown menu.

        i.   /EMMEANS=TABLES(Mode_of_Exercise*EMG_Amplitude) COMPARE(Mode_of_Exercise) ADJ(BONFERRONI).

           1.   This will allow us to examine mean differences between each mode of exercise for each of the three muscles.

        ii.   /EMMEANS=TABLES(Mode_of_Exercise*EMG_Amplitude) COMPARE(EMG_Amplitude) ADJ(BONFERRONI).

           1.   This will allow us to examine mean differences between the three muscles for each mode of exercise.

    c.   After typing the above /EMMEANS syntax, press the green ▶ button to perform the statistical analysis.

Syntax for SPSS for example 2

```
GLM Peak_EMG_Amplitude_VL Peak_EMG_Amplitude_RF Peak_EMG_Amplitude_
VM BY Mode_of_Exercise
/WSFACTOR=EMG_Amplitude 3 Polynomial
/METHOD=SSTYPE(3)
/PLOT=PROFILE(EMG_Amplitude*Mode_of_Exercise)
/EMMEANS=TABLES(Mode_of_Exercise) COMPARE ADJ(BONFERRONI)
/EMMEANS=TABLES(EMG_Amplitude) COMPARE ADJ(BONFERRONI)
/EMMEANS=TABLES(Mode_of_Exercise*EMG_Amplitude) COMPARE(Mode_of_
Exercise) ADJ(BONFERRONI)
/PRINT=DESCRIPTIVE
/CRITERIA=ALPHA(.05)
/WSDESIGN=EMG_Amplitude
/DESIGN=Mode_of_Exercise.
```

Interpreting the output for SPSS for example 2

As shown in Table 5.8, SPSS generates the Within-Subjects Factors table which are the three muscles (vastus lateralis #1, rectus femoris #2, and vastus medialis #3), whereas the Between-Subjects Factors table indicates the two modes of exercise (treadmill running and cycle ergometry). Therefore, the electromyographic (EMG) amplitude was measured from the three muscles during treadmill running as well as cycle ergometry for all subjects.

As shown in Table 5.9, the Mauchly's Test of Sphericity table indicates that we have not met this assumption since the test is statistically significant (*p*-value is 0.042).

As shown in Table 5.10, the Tests of Between-Subjects Effects indicates that there is a main effect for EMG amplitude (i.e., muscles) and a significant interaction. Due to the significant Mauchly's Test of Sphericity the investigator would use the "Greenhouse-Geisser" row to determine significance rather than the "Sphericity Assumed" row.

As shown in Table 5.11, the Tests of Between-Subjects Effect indicates that there was no main effect for mode of exercise.

As shown in Table 5.12, prior to the results of the pairwise comparisons SPSS provides the mean and standard error values for each group and muscle. These are the values to use in when writing your results and/or generating graphs/tables.

Table 5.8 Within-subjects factors, reprint courtesy of International Business Machines Corporation

Within-Subjects Factors
Measure: MEASURE_1

EMG_Amplitude	Dependent variable
1	Peak_EMG_Amplitude_VL
2	Peak_EMG_Amplitude_RF
3	Peak_EMG_Amplitude_VM

Within-Subjects Factors

		Value label	N
Mode_of_Exercise	**.00**	Treadmill	8
	1.00	Cycle Ergometry	7

Source: © International Business Machines Corporation.

Table 5.9 Mauchly's test of sphericity, reprint courtesy of International Business Machines Corporation

Mauchly's Test of Sphericity[a]
Measure: MEASURE_1

Within subjects effect	Mauchly's W	Approx. Chi-Square	df	Sig.	Epsilon[b] Greenhouse-Geisser	Hunh-Feldt	Lower-bound
EMG_Amplitude	.590	6.327	2	.042	.709	.832	.500

Source: © International Business Machines Corporation.

Notes
Tests the null hypothesis that the error covariance matrix of the orthonormalized transformed dependent variables is proportional to an identity matrix.
a Design: Intercept + Mode_of_Exercise.
  Within Subjects Design: EMG_Amplitude
b May be used to adjust the degrees of freedom for the averaged tests of significance. Corrected tests are displayed in the Tests of Within-Subjects Effects table.

Table 5.10 Tests of within-subjects effects, reprint courtesy of International Business Machines Corporation

Tests of Within-Subjects Effects
Measure: MEASURE_1

Source		Type III sum of squares	df.	Mean square	F	Sig.
EMG_Amplitude	Spherically Assumed	87405.854	2	43702.927	61.933	.000
	Greenhouse_Geisser	87405.854	1.419	61611.943	61.933	.000
	Huynh-Feldt	87405.854	1.665	52504.664	61.933	.000
	Lower-bound	87405.854	1.000	87405.854	61.933	.000
EMG_Amplitude*Mode_of_Exercise	Spherically Assumed	25795.309	2	12897.655	18.278	.000
	Greenhouse_Geisser	25795.309	1.419	18182.983	18.278	.000
	Huynh-Feldt	25795.309	1.665	15495.232	18.278	.000
	Lower-bound	25795.309	1.000	25795.309	18.278	.000
Error(EMG_Amplitude)	Spherically Assumed	18346.844	26	705.648		
	Greenhouse_Geisser	18346.844	18.442	994.815		
	Huynh-Feldt	18346.844	21.641	847.765		
	Lower-bound	18346.844	13.000	1411.296		

Source: © International Business Machines Corporation.

Table 5.11 Tests of between-subjects effects, reprint courtesy of International Business Machines Corporation

Tests of Between-Subjects Effects
Measure: MEASURE_1
Transformed Variable: Average

Source	Type III sum of squares	df.	Mean square	F	Sig.
Intercept	2293771.659	1	229771.659	213.478	.000
Mode_of_Exercise	35038.905	1	35038.905	3.261	**.0.94**
Error	139681.851	13	10744.758		

Source: © International Business Machines Corporation.

Table 5.12 Estimates, reprint courtesy of International Business Machines Corporation

Estimates
Measure: MEASURE_1

Mode_of_ Exercise	EMG_ Amplitude	Mean	Std. error	95% confidence interval	
				Lower bound	Upper bound
Treadmill	VL	319.040	19.870	276.114	361.967
	RF	264.337	23.702	213.131	315.543
	VM	179.346	23.725	128.091	230.601
Cycle Ergometry	VL	195.986	21.242	150.095	241.876
	RF	250.668	25.339	195.927	305.410
	VM	148.271	25.363	93.477	203.064

Source: © International Business Machines Corporation.

Table 5.13 Univariate tests, reprint courtesy of International Business Machines Corporation

Univariate Tests
Measure: MEASURE_1

EMG_Amplitude		Sum of squares	df.	Mean square	F	Sig.
1	Contrast	56531.522	1	56531.522	17.898	.001
	Error	41061.270	13	3158.559		
2	Contrast	597.502	1	697.502	.155	.700
	Error	584.044	13	4494.465		
3	Contrast	3605.190	1	3605.190	.801	.387
	Error	58539.380	13	4503.029		

Source: © International Business Machines Corporation.

Note
Each F tests the simple effects of Mode_of_Exercise within each level combination of the other effects shown. These tests are based on the linearly independent pairwise comparisons among the estimated marginal means.

Table 5.14 Pairwise comparisons, reprint courtesy of International Business Machines Corporation

Pairwise Comparisons
Measure: MEASURE_1

EMG_Amplitude	(I) Mode_of_Exercise	(J) Mode_of_Exercise	Mean difference (I–J)	Std. error	Sig.[b]	95% confidence interval for difference[b]	
						Lower bound	Upper bound
1	Treadmill	Cycle Ergometry	123.054	29.087	.001	60.216	185.893
	Cycle Ergometry	Treadmill	−123.054*	29.087	.001	−185.893	−60.216
2	Treadmill	Cycle Ergometry	13.669	34.697	.700	−61.289	88.627
	Cycle Ergometry	Treadmill	−13.669	34.697	.700	−88.627	61.289
3	Treadmill	Cycle Ergometry	31.075	34.730	.387	−43.954	106.105
	Cycle Ergometry	Treadmill	−31.075	34.730	.387	−106.105	43.954

Source: © International Business Machines Corporation.

Notes
Based on estimated marginal means.
* The mean difference is significant at the .05 level.
b Adjustment for multiple comparisons: Bonferroni.

As shown in Table 5.13, the Univariate Tests table is generated which indicates that there was a significant overall *F*-ratio for the first muscle (vastus lateralis).

As shown in Table 5.14, the Pairwise Comparisons table shows that for the first muscle (vastus lateralis), there are significant mean differences between the two modes of exercise. Keep in mind that this table was generated from the /EMMEANS=TABLES(Mode_of_Exercise*EMG_Amplitude)   COMPARE(Mode_of_Exercise) ADJ(BONFERRONI) syntax line.

Sample write-up for example 2

The 2×3 mixed factorial ANOVA revealed a significant interaction [$F(1.4,18.4)=18.278$; $p<0.001$] and a significant main effect for EMG amplitude [$F(1.4,18.4)=61.9$; $p<0.001$], but not a significant main effect for mode [$F(1,13)=3.261$; $p=0.094$]. For the follow-up test we examined mean differences in EMG amplitude between treadmill exercise and cycle ergometry for each muscle. For the VL muscle, therefore, we found significant mean differences (treadmill: $319\pm20\mu$Vrms vs. cycle ergometry: $196\pm21\mu$Vrms; $p=0.01$), but no significant mean differences between modes for the rectus femoris (treadmill: $264\pm23\mu$Vrms vs. cycle ergometry: $251\pm25\mu$Vrms; $p=0.700$) and vastus medialis (treadmill: $179\pm24\mu$Vrms vs. cycle ergometry: $148\pm25\mu$Vrms; $p=0.387$) muscles.

6 Analysis of covariance (ANCOVA)

Introduction

Scientists want to account for factors other than the independent variable which may influence their dependent variable. For example, if the investigator is examining muscular strength in young adults their inclusion criteria may restrict participants to those who are between 20 and 30 years old and, therefore, the investigator would exclude anyone outside this age range. There are situations, however, in which the investigator may not be able to control for certain factors. For example, the investigator may be conducting a study which examines the effects of caffeine on endurance performance, yet most people consume some amount of caffeine daily. So what does the investigator do? One option may be to have each subject complete a caffeine consumption questionnaire and then statistically adjust for the effects of caffeine consumption in their analysis. As a result, the investigator has to use daily caffeine consumption as a covariate thus reducing the error variability in their study. This type of statistical procedure is called Analysis of Covariance (ANCOVA).

ANCOVA **should not** be used arbitrarily to replace a sloppy research design which lacks the appropriate experimental control. Therefore, a strong justification needs to be presented for why each covariate is going to be used. In addition, the use of multiple covariates is not advisable (i.e., more than three), because it makes the interpretation of the results more complex.

Research questions

The types of research questions for ANCOVA are similar to studies we have already described in previous ANOVA chapters. The difference here, however, is that there may be a variable which is influencing the dependent variable and that is difficult or impossible to control. It is important to reiterate that the implementation of ANCOVA should be used judiciously with strong justification. For example, if the investigator wanted to study upper body strength on a group of volleyball players, they might assume that the player's strength would be related, in part, to any strength training regimen the athlete has been performing. In this case, the investigator would ask each subject a question such as, "*In the last 6 months, how many hours per week have you lifted weights for your upper body?*" This information, therefore, will provide the investigator an index of each subject's upper body strength training regimen. That is, since the investigator is interested in measuring upper body strength, they do not want the athlete's past (or current) training regimen to influence the results by adding more variability (i.e., error) to the dependent variable.

Review of ANCOVA

ANCOVA works by "holding constant" the covariate across group means. That is, for a dependent variable, each group mean has the variance associated with the covariate accounted for in the model separately, so that all group means adjusted for the influence of the covariate. This "new" mean for each group is called the *adjusted group mean*.

The assumptions of ANOVA (*see previous chapters*) apply to ANCOVA with two additional assumptions. First, we need to make sure that there is a linear relationship between the dependent variable and the covariate. This is critical, because the adjusted means are derived from linear regression and, therefore, if the relationship between the dependent variable and covariate is curvilinear then adjusted means will be invalid. A simple approach to determining if there is a linear relationship between the dependent variable and covariate is to create a scatterplot to visually inspect the relationship. A second assumption of ANCOVA is homogeneity of regression. The purpose of this assumption is to determine if all groups have similar regression slopes (i.e., similar direction) for the dependent variable and covariate. The assumption when met assumes that adjustment to the dependent variable by the covariate is in the same direction for each independent variable group. Ideally, the investigator would want the slopes to be the same for all groups. If, however, this assumption is violated, then ANCOVA cannot be used, and an alternative approach would need to be implemented.

It is important to note that for ANCOVA, a Type I Sum of Squares decomposition needs to be requested. Typically, in ANOVA-based designs, a Type III Sum of Squares decomposition is evaluated to provide an unweighted means analysis of your design (accounting possible unequal cell sizes which might lead to a condition effect in factorial designs), which simultaneously adjusts effects in your model for all other effects. But in ANCOVA, we wish to remove the effects of the covariate first, followed by the effect(s) of interest. This provides an appropriate test of the covariate unadjusted for the independent variable(s) in your model, and then provides the independent variable effect(s) adjusted for the covariate. Therefore, in SPSS you need to purposely select a Type I Sum of Squares in the "Model" window.

Example of one-way ANCOVA (example 1)

Provided in this first example is a straightforward illustration of performing ANCOVA. In this generic example, there are two groups (control and experimental), a covariate, and the dependent variable. More complex designs of ANCOVA can be built on this basic example. When performing an ANCOVA, and in addition to the assumptions noted in the ANOVA chapter, you must first determine if the HOR (homogeneity of regression) assumption is met.

Using SPSS pulldown menu for HOR analysis (example 1)

1. Click **Analyze**, then click **General Linear Model**, then click **Univariate.**
2. Click **Group** and move to Fixed Factor(s).
3. Next, click **dependent_variable** and move to Dependent Variable.
4. Then click **Covariate** and move to Covariate(s).
5. Click **Model**, then click **Custom** (*in newer versions of SPSS this is labeled "Build terms"*).

    a. Click **Group** and move to Model Column.

    b. Then click **Covariate** and move to Model Column.

    c. Next, click both **Group** and **Covariate** (*by holding the Shift key*) and move to Model column.

    d. Change Sum of squares from Type III to Type I and then click **Continue.**

6. Click **OK.**

Syntax for HOR analysis (example 1)

```
UNIANOVA dependent_variable BY Group WITH covariate
/METHOD=SSTYPE(1)
/INTERCEPT=INCLUDE
/CRITERIA=ALPHA(0.05)
/DESIGN=covariate Group covariate*Group.
```

Interpreting the output for HOR analysis (example 1)

As shown in Table 6.1, for the HOR analysis SPSS generates the Tests of Between-Subjects Effects table. The group × covariate interaction, which is what we wish to focus upon, is not statistically significant ($p = 0.833$). Thus, we can conclude that the HOR assumption was met and therefore use the covariate in the ANCOVA analysis.

Table 6.1 Tests of between-subject effects, reprint courtesy of International Business Machines Corporation.

Tests of Between-Subjects Effects
Dependent Variable: dependent_variable

Source	Type I sum of squares	df.	Mean square	F	Sig.
Corrected Model	93883.623[a]	3	31294.541	10.246	.024
Intercept	799949.956	1	799949.956	261.917	.000
Covariate	22787.817	1	22787.817	7.461	.052
Group	70941.492	1	70941.492	23.227	.009
Group*covariate	154.314	1	154.314	.051	.833
Error	12216.859	1	3054.215		
Total	906050.438	8			
Corrected Total	106100.482	7			

Source: © International Business Machines Corporation.

Note
a R Squared = .885 (Adjusted R Squared = .798).

Using SPSS pulldown menu for ANCOVA analysis after meeting HOR assumption (example 1)

1. Click **Analyze**, then click **General Linear Model**, then click **Univariate.**
2. Click **Reset** to discard the previous HOR analysis.
3. Click **Group** and move to Fixed Factor(s), then click **dependent_variable** and move to Dependent Variable, then click **Covariate** and move to Covariate(s).

   a.   Click **Model.**
   b.   Change Sum of squares from Type III to Type I and then click **Continue.**

4. Click **Options**, then click **GROUP** and move to "Display means for" box.

   a.   then check the **Descriptive statistics** box, then click **Continue.**

5. Click **OK.**

Syntax for ANCOVA after meeting HOR assumption (example 1)

UNIANOVA dependent_variable BY Group WITH covariate
/METHOD=SSTYPE(1)
/INTERCEPT=INCLUDE
/PLOT=PROFILE(Group)
/EMMEANS=TABLES(Group) WITH(covariate=MEAN)
/PRINT=DESCRIPTIVE
/CRITERIA=ALPHA(.05)
/DESIGN=covariate Group.

Interpreting the output for SPSS after meeting HOR assumption (example 1)

As shown in Table 6.2, the Tests of Between-Subjects Effects generated by SPSS there is a significant effect for the group factor ($p = 0.003$). In Table 6.3, SPSS produces the mean and standard error values for the control and experimental groups. It is important to note, that these mean values have been adjusted for the covariate as indicated at the bottom of Table 6.3.

Table 6.2 Tests of between-subjects effects, reprint courtesy of International Business Machines Corporation

Tests of Between-Subjects Effects
Dependent Variable: dependent_variable

Source	Type I sum of squares	df.	Mean square	F	Sig.
Corrected Model	93729.309[a]	2	46864.654	18.941	.005
Intercept	799949.956	1	799949.956	323.312	.000
Covariate	22787.817	1	22787.817	9.210	.029
Group	70941.492	1	70941.492	28.672	.003
Error	12371.173	5	2474.235		
Total	906050.438	8			
Corrected Total	106100.482	7			

Source: © International Business Machines Corporation.

Note
a R Squared = .883 (Adjusted R Squared = .837).

Table 6.3 Group, reprint courtesy of International Business Machines Corporation

Group

Dependent Variable: dependent_variable

Group	Mean	Std. error	95% confidence interval	
			Lower bound	Upper bound
Control	410.41[a]	24.87	346.47	474.36
Exp.	222.02[a]	24.87	158.08	285.96

Source: © International Business Machines Corporation.

Note

a Covariates appearing in the model are evaluated at the following values: covariate = 65.62500.

Sample write-up (example 1)

A one-way ANCOVA was performed in the current investigation. Prior to the main analysis, the homogeneity of regression (HOR) assumption was assessed and found to be tenable; the interaction of the independent variable and the covariate was not significant, $F(1,4) = 0.051$, $p = 0.833$, indicating parallel slope adjustment on the dependent variable for levels of our independent variable. The ANCOVA analysis revealed a significant overall F-ratio [$F(1,5) = 28.67$, $p = 0.003$]. Thus, there was a significant mean difference between the two groups [410 ± 25 vs. 222 ± 25; $p = 0.003$].

Example of two-way ANCOVA (example 2)

In this second example, we extend the one-way ANCOVA example from above with some slight modifications. Specifically, for the group variable we now have three levels (control, placebo, or experimental) and we have added a second factor (fitness level) which has three levels (sedentary, active, or highly active). When performing a two-way ANCOVA, you must first determine if the HOR (homogeneity of regression) assumption is met.

Using SPSS pulldown menu for HOR analysis (example 2)

1. Click **Analyze**, then click **General Linear Model**, then click **Univariate**.
2. Hold the Shift key and then click **Group** and **Fitness_Level** and then move to Fixed Factor(s).
3. Next, click **dependent_variable** and move to Dependent Variable.
4. Then click **Covariate** and move to Covariate(s).
5. Click **Model**, then click **Custom** (*in newer versions of SPSS it may be labelled "Build terms"*).

   a. Holding the Shift key, click **Group** and **Fitness_Level** and then move to Model Column.
   b. Holding the Shift key, click **Group** and **Covariate** and then move to Model Column.
   c. Holding the Shift key, click **Fitness_Level** and **Covariate** and then move to Model Column.

    d.   Holding the Shift key, click **Group, Fitness_Level,** and **Covariate** and then move to Model Column.

    e.   Change Sum of squares from Type III to Type I and then click **Continue.**

6.   Click **OK.**

Syntax for HOR analysis (example 2, two-way ANCOVA)[1]

UNIANOVA dependent_variable BY Group Fitness_Level WITH covariate
/METHOD=SSTYPE(1)
/INTERCEPT=INCLUDE
/CRITERIA=ALPHA(0.05)
/DESIGN=covariate, Group, Fitness_Level, Group*Fitness_Level,
covariate*Group, covariate*Fitness_Level, covariate*Group*Fitness_Level.

Interpreting the output for HOR analysis (example 2, two-way ANCOVA)

As shown in Table 6.4, for the HOR analysis SPSS generates the Tests of Between-Subjects Effects table. The points of emphasis are the various interaction terms within the table. In all four cases, the interaction terms are not significant (*p*-values ranging from 0.221 to 0.903). Thus, the HOR assumption was met.

Using SPSS pulldown menu for ANCOVA analysis after meeting HOR assumption (example 2)

1.   Click **Analyze,** then click **General Linear Model,** then click **Univariate.**
2.   Click **Reset** to discard the previous HOR analysis.

Table 6.4 Tests of between-subjects effects, reprint courtesy of International Business Machines Corporation

Tests of Between-Subjects Effects
Dependent Variable: dependent_variable

Source	Type I sum of squares	df.	Mean square	F	Sig.
Corrected Model	34858.185	11	3168.926	.957	.487
Intercept	17307197.78	1	17307197.78	5227.215	.000
Covariate	10333.957	1	10333.957	3.121	.079
Group	1918.111	2	959.056	.290	.749
Fitness_Level	2676.935	2	1338.468	.404	.668
Group*Fitness_Level	7410.799	1	7410.799	2.238	.136
Group*covariate	3171.432	2	1585.716	.479	.620
Fitness_Level*covariate	9298.042	2	4649.021	1.404	.248
Group*Fitness_Level*covariate	48.907	1	48.907	.015	.903
Error	622464.035	188	3310.979		
Total	17964520.00	200			
Corrected Total	657322.220	199			

Source: © International Business Machines Corporation.

3. Hold down the Shift key and click on **Group** and **Fitness_Level** then move to Fixed Factor(s).
4. Then click **dependent_variable** and move to Dependent Variable, then click **Covariate** and move to Covariate(s).

   a. Click **Model**.
   b. Change Sum of squares from Type III to Type I and then click **Continue**.

5. Click **Options**.

   a. Then click **GROUP** and move to "Display means for" box.
   b. Then click **Fitness_Level** and move to "Display means for" box.
   c. Then click **GROUP* Fitness_Level** and move to "Display means for" box.
   d. Click the box next to Compare main effects.
   i. From the pulldown menu select Bonferroni.
   e. Check the **Descriptive statistics** box.
   f. Then click **Continue**.

6. Click **OK**.

Syntax for ANCOVA after meeting HOR assumption (example 2, Two-way ANOVA)

UNIANOVA dependent_variable BY Group Fitness_Level WITH covariate
/METHOD=SSTYPE(1)
/INTERCEPT=INCLUDE
/EMMEANS=TABLES(Group)   WITH(covariate=MEAN)   COMPARE   ADJ (BONFERRONI)
/EMMEANS=TABLES(Fitness_Level) WITH(covariate=MEAN) COMPARE ADJ (BONFERRONI)
/EMMEANS=TABLES(Group*Fitness_Level) WITH(covariate=MEAN)
/PRINT DESCRIPTIVE
/CRITERIA=ALPHA(.05)
/DESIGN=covariate Group Fitness_Level Group*Fitness_Level.

Interpreting the output for SPSS after meeting the HOR assumption (example 2, two-way ANCOVA)

As shown in Table 6.5, the Between-Subjects Factors generated by SPSS shows the two factors (group and fitness level) as well as their corresponding levels and label for each of those levels.

In Table 6.6, SPSS produces the Tests of Between-Subjects Effects table which will indicate whether or not there are significant main effects for group and fitness level as well as a significant interaction term when using the covariate variable. In this example, the p-value for the interaction term (group × fitness level) is not statistically significant ($p = 0.135$). Moreover, the p-values for the group and fitness level main effects are $p = 0.747$ and $p = 0.666$, respectively. Thus, there are also no significant main effects. Due to the lack of significant findings, no *post-hoc* testing is required.

Table 6.5 Between-subject factors, reprint courtesy of International Business Machines Corporation

Between-Subjects Factors

		Value label	N
Group	0	Control	76
	1	Placebo	44
	2	Experimental	80
Fitness_Level	1	Sedentary	86
	2	Active	67
	3	Highly Active	37

Source: © International Business Machines Corporation.

Table 6.6 Tests of between-subjects effects, reprint courtesy of International Business Machines Corporation

Tests of Between-Subjects Effects
Dependent Variable: dependent_variable

Source	Type I sum of squares	df.	Mean square	F	Sig.
Corrected Model	22339.804[a]	6	3723.301	1.132	.345
Intercept	17307197.78	1	17307197.78	5227.215	.000
covariate	10333.957	1	10333.957	3.141	.078
Group	1918.111	2	959.056	.292	.747
Fitness_Level	2676.935	2	1338.468	.407	.666
Group*Fitness_Level	7410.799	1	7410.799	2.252	.135
Error	634982.416	193	3290.064		
Total	17964520.00	200			
Corrected Total	657322.220	199			

Source: © International Business Machines Corporation.

Note
a R Squared = .034 (Adjusted R Squared = .004).

Sample write-up (example 2, two-way ANCOVA)

The two-way ANCOVA was performed in the present study. Prior to the formal analysis, an evaluation of the homogeneity of regression (HOR) assumption was performed. None of the covariate interactions were significant and, therefore it was concluded that the HOR assumption was met. The formal 3 [group: control, placebo, or experimental] × 3 [fitness level: sedentary, active, or highly active] ANCOVA revealed no significant interaction [$F(1,193) = 2.252$; $p = 0.135$]. Moreover, there were no significant main effects for group [$F(2,193) = 0.292$; $p = 0.747$] or fitness level [$F(2,193) = 0.407$; $p = 0.666$]. Due to the lack of any significant findings, we failed to reject the null hypothesis.

Note

1. An alternative method to assess HOR in factorial ANCOVA is to use the MANOVA syntax in SPSS, which will give a single grouped interaction term for all independent variables and the covariate. The syntax below illustrates this approach:

```
MANOVA dependent_variable BY Group (0,2) Fitness_Level (1,3) WITH covariate
/print = signif(brief)
/analysis = dv
/method=sequential
/design covariate Group Fitness_Level Group*Fitness_Level
covariate*Group+covariate*Fitness_Level+covariate*Group*Fitness_Level.
```

Part II
Regression analysis

7   Diagnostic tests for regression

Introduction

After completing data collection and prior to beginning the formal regression analyses, it is incumbent on the investigator to screen their data. Typically, this process is called data cleaning in which the investigator examines each variable in the data set to assure that errors have not been made. Errors can range from simple typographic mistakes such as transcribing the subject's weight in pounds when in fact kilograms were the units needed, to errors which may not be initially or readily obvious and can potentially skew the results of your formal statistical analyses. Therefore, the present chapter will focus on this latter error by introducing established data screening procedures used to identify outliers within a given data set.

Review of regression assumptions

As discussed in the ANOVA section, quantitative models have assumptions which first need to be met in order to generate valid conclusions about the population of interest. Similarly, regression analysis has its own set of assumptions: (i) normality; (ii) linearity; (iii) homoscedasticity; (iv) multicollinearity; and (v) independence.

Normality. Normality refers the data for each variable having a normal distribution and not being skewed in one direction or another.

Linearity. Linearity, as named, refers to the linear relationship amongst the independent and dependent variables. Therefore, if data are curvilinear then any predictions from a linear model may be biased. Linearity may be detected through bivariate scatterplots and evaluating whether the plotted points create a straight-line association. The observed versus the predicted values may also be plotted, which will result in a scatterplot with the data points distributed around the regression line.

Homoscedasticity. Homoscedasticity indicates that the variation for the residuals is constant without noticeable patterns. That is, the variances of the dependent variable at the various levels of the independent variable are approximately equal. To determine if the homoscedasticity assumption has been violated (i.e., heteroscedasticity), plot the residuals versus the predicted values. The plotted values should be equally distributed along the zero point forming a rough rectangle. Violation of homoscedasticity would be indicated by the plotted values flaring in or out (> or <) like a sieve. Note that this assessment (plotting the residuals vs. predicted values) can also be used to assess multivariate normality and linearity.

Multicollinearity. Multicollinearity refers to extremely high correlations (usually 0.90 or above) between predictors, or between predictors and the criterion. Correlations of 0.90 or higher between variables can be problematic causing strange analytical results – for example, extreme standard errors thus producing Type II errors in significance of predictors. Variables correlated at 0.90 or higher may be deemed "the same" variable essentially, since the overlapping variance is at least 81 percent. That being said, research in the medical sciences and related fields may indeed find variables so highly correlated are important to include in the regression since medical and health outcomes are highly determined or influenced by biological markers. If the researcher deems multicollinearity to be problematic, consider dropping one of the variables. Assessment of multicollinearity is done by evaluating the bivariate correlation matrix between variables and criterion. Also, *tolerance* may be assessed, which is 1 minus the squared multiple correlation (SMC) of a predictor by the other predictors in the regression (1 – SMC). Extremely low tolerance values such as 0.10 can indicate high multicollinearity, although values <0.20 may also be of concern. The *variance inflation factor* (VIF) may also be assessed, calculated as 1/tolerance. Values greater than 10 suggest high multicollinearity, and if the average of the VIF values across variables exceeds 1.0, that is also indicative of problematic multicollinearity.

Independence. Independence refers to the independence of errors in the prediction of the criterion. Nonindependence of errors of prediction suggests there is some dependency between the order of cases in the data and the regression variables. One example of such a dependency bias would be "time," where due to interviewer effects those sampled earlier during the study period show more varied responses compared to those later sampled. Violation of this assumption can be assessed by plotting the residuals by the order cases were assessed. A formal test of this assumption is the *Durbin-Watson test*, which looks at the autocorrelation of errors by the case sequence. The Durbin-Watson test ranges between 0 and 4, with values close to 2 indicating uncorrelated errors (values close to 0 or 4 indicate extreme positive or negative autocorrelation, respectively). Values between 1.5 and 2.5 are indicative of independence.

Identifying outliers

It is essential prior to performing your formal statistical analyses to screen your data. This is important because it will assist in identifying case(s) that are outliers. An outlier may be a data point with an extremely higher or lower value related to other data points for that variable. Outliers may be simple typographical errors (such as entering the number 500 when you meant to enter 50) or more complex. Nevertheless, it is important to remember that outliers may potentially distort the results of your formal test statistic. A number of different data screening techniques are used to identify outliers.

Bivariate plots. Bivariate scatterplots of the predictors and the criterion can reveal cases that across pairs of variables have extreme high or low values. Cases that fall outside the "swarm" of values in these plots may be outliers and should be evaluated further for adjustment or exclusion. It may be assessed through bivariate plots of the predictors, and is revealed by looking for cases that are removed from the swarm of plotted values. As a general example, say two variables (age and income) are used to predict a measure of community status. Focusing on age and income, someone who is 18 years of age might be typical in a community sample, as would someone making $100,000 per year. A bivariate plot of these data might reveal an 18 year old who earns $100,000 per year – such a case may be considered high in leverage if it appears removed or separate from the other plotted values.

Standardized residuals (ZRESID). The ZRESID are expressed on the z-score scale and are calculated by dividing the residual $(Y_i - Y)$ by the standard deviation of the sample deviations. A large standardized residual indicates a case is ill-fit by the regression line and may be an outlier.

Adjusted predicted value (ADJPRED). The ADJPRED is the adjusted predicted value, where the predicted value from the regression equation is calculated removing the *i*th case $(Y' = a + b_i^{(i)} x_i)$, where (i) indicates the removal of the *i*th case. If the ADJPRED is noticeably different from the original predicted value, the *i*th case may be an outlier.

Deleted residuals (DRESID) and studentized deleted residuals (SDRESID). The DRESID is the deleted residual, which is a recalculation of the residuals with the *i*th case removed $(Y_i - Y'^{(i)}_i)$. If the DRESID is noticeably different from the calculated residual, then the case may be overly influential. The SDRESID is the studentized deleted residual, which is calculated by taking the deleted residual and dividing it by its standard error. As with the DRESID, if the SDRESID is noticeably different from the SRESID (the studentized residual), then the case may be overly influential.

Influential data point

Leverage. Leverage reflects a case that may be considered distant from other cases across the predictors or independent variables. Leverage is not inclusive of the dependent variable, but instead focuses on the independent variables or predictors. Formal calculations to assess leverage are offered in various statistical programs, with leverage values ranging from 0 to 1. The resulting values may be compared to a cutoff value – if a leverage value exceeds the cutoff, the case may have undue influence on the resulting regression line. The cutoff value is calculated as follows (with k indicating the number of predictors in the regression model):

$$2\left(\frac{k+1}{N}\right)$$ **Formula 10.1 Leverage cutoff value**

Cook's distance (Cook's D). Influence and its resulting assessment using Cook's distance (Cook's D) also reflects a case's influence on the regression line. It is a measure of change in the residuals when the *i*th case is removed. Although one can simply note the difference between the residual and the deleted residual for a given case to provide an assessment of a case's influence, Cook's D provides a broader look since it encompasses change in all of the residuals. Larger values of Cook's D indicate greater case influence. A rough cutoff to indicate the case may be problematic can be calculated using $4/(N-2)$, with N being the total number of cases. If Cook's D for a case exceeds the cutoff, it may have an undue influence on the regression line.

$$C_i = \frac{\sum (Y'^{(i)} - Y')^2}{(p+1)S^2}$$ **Formula 10.2 Cook's distance**

Research question

The investigator is interested in performing diagnostics on the regression model they are planning to develop. Below we present the interpretations of the various methods of screening the data set. Thereafter, we present the pulldown menu instructions and syntax commands for achieving each analyses.

Interpretation of data screening

Normality, linearity, and homoscedasticity

In starting to make our assessment, we begin by assessing *normality*. This is done by evaluating histograms of the variables in the planned regression, and is considered a univariate or single variable assessment (a multivariate normality assessment will be covered shortly). Figures 7.1 and 7.2 illustrate the syntax and resulting histogram for two of the variables (oxygen uptake and age). Keep in mind that the criterion variable is oxygen uptake and will be referred to as such in the examples below. For both histograms, a slight skew is noted, but in general it may be concluded that these variables are approximately normal.

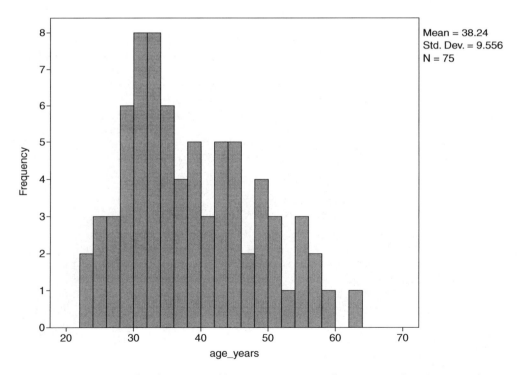

Figure 7.1 Histogram for the age variable, reprint courtesy of International Business Machines Corporation.

Source: © International Business Machines Corporation.

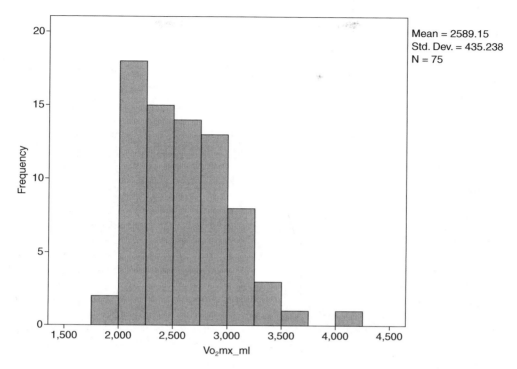

Figure 7.2 Histogram for V̇o₂ *max* variable, reprint courtesy of International Business Machines Corporation.

Source: © International Business Machines Corporation.

Next, we assess *linearity* using bivariate scatterplots which is performed for all variables in the planned regression. In Figure 7.3, we present syntax for the bivariate plots of the criterion with age, and with weight. In these graphs, we wish to see straight-line associations (an absence of curvilinearity). Although not perfectly aligned, the graphs suggest linearity is tenable. Since these are bivariate assessments, a multivariate assessment should also be performed (to be demonstrated in the next section).

Homoscedasticity is assessed by plotting the standardized predicted values by standardized residuals. This same multivariate plot is also used to assess multivariate normality and linearity. To assess homoscedasticity (and multivariate normality and linearity), run the planned regression analysis and request a plot of the standardized predicted values by the standardized residuals. This is demonstrated in Figure 7.4. To meet all three multivariate assumptions, the plotted values should be equally distributed along the zero point forming a rough rectangle. Violation of homoscedasticity would be indicated by the plotted values flaring in or out (> or <) like a sieve. Violation of normality would be indicated by the plotted cases clustered either below or above the zero mark (as opposed to being equally distributed). Violation of linearity would be indicated by the plotted cases forming a ∪ or ∩ association thereby suggesting a curved association. In Figure 7.4, the cases meet the assumptions of

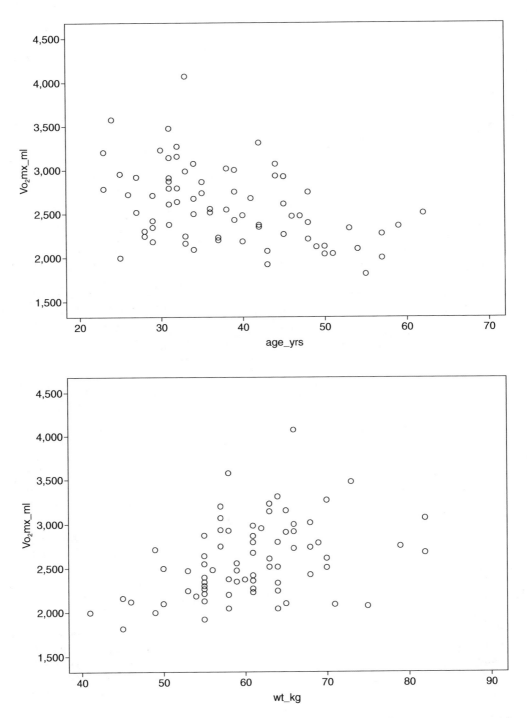

Figure 7.3 Bivariate plots of the criterion with age and weight variables, reprint courtesy of International Business Machines Corporation.

Source: © International Business Machines Corporation.

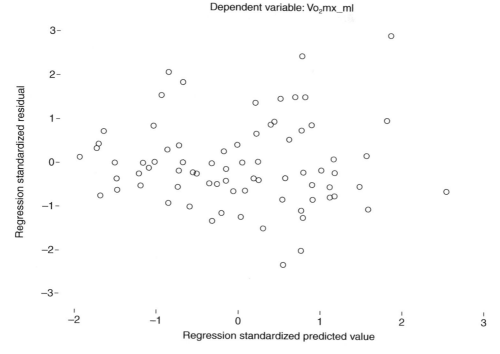

Figure 7.4 Homoscedasticity plot scatterplot, reprint courtesy of International Business Machines Corporation.

Source: © International Business machines corporation.

multivariate normality and linearity. However, there may be an issue with homoscedasticity since the plotted cases flare outward (<), which may produce a degraded solution and thus increase the likelihood of Type II error.

The graph above (Figure 7.4) illustrates a fairly good spread of the standardized residuals plotted against standardized predicted values. If we draw a horizontal line at the zero point along the ordinal axis (regression standardized residual), the plot points equally fall above/below the line, suggesting multivariate normality. Using this same horizontal line, we may also assess homoscedasticity. Here, the plot points generally fall above/below the line, although there is a slight flaring pattern suggesting heteroscedasticity, which may produce a degraded solution. Thus, borderline regression results should be interpreted carefully. If we next draw a line of best fit across the plot points, there appears to be a straight-line association (no clear curvilinear association), suggesting multivariate linearity.

Multicollinearity is assessed using bivariate correlations, tolerance, and the variance inflation factor (VIF). Bivariate correlations are presented in Table 7.1, with tolerance and the VIF presented in Table 7.2. None of the bivariate correlations across variables exceed 0.90. The tolerance values are well above 0.10, and the VIF values well below 10 (with the average VIF exceeding 1.0 as well). Extreme multicollinearity does not appear to be an issue within our data.

Table 7.1 Correlations, reprint courtesy of International Business Machines Corporation

Correlations

		Vo2mx_ml	wt_kg	ht_meter	age_yrs	Times/wk_exercise	Intensity of subjects training (6–20)
Vo2mx_ml	Pearson Correlation	1	.413	.577	-.442	.216	.373
	Sig. (2-tailed)		.000	.000	.000	.063	.001
	N	75	75	75	75	75	75
wt_kg	Pearson Correlation	.413	1	.599	-.058	.069	-.197
	Sig. (2-tailed)	.000		.000	.624	.554	.091
	N	75	75	75	75	75	75
ht_meter	Pearson Correlation	.577	.599	2	-.331	.144	.062
	Sig. (2-tailed)	.000	.000		.004	.216	.594
	N	75	75	75	75	75	75
age_yrs	Pearson Correlation	-.442	-.058	-.331	.1	-.134	-.139
	Sig. (2-tailed)	.000	.624	.004		.252	.236
	N	75	75	75	75	75	75
Times/wk_exercise	Pearson Correlation	.216	.069	.144	-.134	1	.206
	Sig. (2-tailed)	.063	.554	.216	.252		.077
	N	75	75	75	75	75	75
Intensity of subjects training (6–20)	Pearson Correlation	.373	-.197	.062	-.139	.206	1
	Sig. (2-tailed)	.001	.091	.594	.236	.077	
	N	75	75	75	75	75	75

Table 7.2 Excluded variables, reprint courtesy of International Business Machines Corporation

Excluded Variables[a]

Model		Beta in	t	Sig.	Partial correlation	Colinearity statistics		
						Tolerance	VIF	Minimum tolerance
1	Times/wk_exercise	.112[b]	1.226	.224	.145	.971	1.030	.549
	Intensity of subjects training (6–20)	.377[b]	4.477	.000	.472	.905	1.105	.533

Source: © International Business Machines Corporation.

Notes
a Dependent Variable: Vo$_2$mx_ml.
b Predictors in the Model: (Constant), age_yrs, wt_kg, ht_meter.

Multicollinearity is assessed in the table above (Table 7.2) focusing on the tolerance and VIF (variance inflation factor). The two statistics are related (1/VIF = tolerance). Low tolerance values (<0.20) suggest possible multicollinearity. For VIF, a single value greater than 10 is problematic, while an "average" VIF across all variables exceeding 1.0 may suggest multicollinearity issues. Evaluating Model 1 above, no variables have tolerance values less than 0.20. For VIF, all values are well below 10, and the average VIF exceeds 1.0. Therefore, there does not appear to be multicollinearity in our model that may bias the regressions results.

Independence of errors of prediction

This is assessed requesting the Durbin-Watson statistic, which tests the assumption of independence of errors of prediction. Table 7.3 contains the necessary syntax to produce the Durbin-Watson statistic. As noted earlier, values between 1.5 and 2.5 are indicative of independence. In our example the Durbin-Watson statistic is 2.082, well within the acceptable range.

As noted earlier, the Durbin-Watson test assesses autocorrelation of errors by the case sequence to evaluate independence of errors. That is, are adjacent case residuals correlated, or independent? As shown in Table 7.3, our value of 2.082 is close to 2.0 (indicative of independence).

Table 7.3 Model summary, reprint courtesy of International Business Machines Corporation

Model Summary[c]

Model	R	R square	Adjusted R square	Std. error of the estimate	Durbin-Watson
1	.650[a]	.422	.398	337.741	
2	.743[b]	.553	.520	301.511	2.082

Source: © International Business Machines Corporation.

Notes
a Predictors: (Constant), age_yrs, wt_kg, ht_meter.
b Predictors: (Constant), age_yrs, wt_kg, ht_meter, Times/wk_exercise, intensity of subjects training (6–20).
c Dependent Variable: Vo$_2$mx_ml.

Outlier assessment

Outliers are assessed through a number of different ways. Bivariate plots (for example, those in Figure 7.2) can be assessed for data points beyond the swarm of plotted points. In Figure 7.3, most cases are reasonable, although a few straggling cases are noted in each plot. The question to ask, however, is whether these straggling cases are indeed outliers and whether they are having an undue influence on the overall regression? Further assessment using additional techniques will help answer this question.

The standardized residuals are also evaluated to assess outliers, along with the adjusted predicted values and deleted residuals. Table 7.4 is the syntax and output to assess the standardized residuals. The most extreme ten cases are printed, and a histogram of the residuals is also presented. Overall, two cases have standardized residuals exceeding ± 2.56 indicating problematic fit. Whether these cases have an undue influence on the regression line will be assessed in a later section, but here we should be at least moderately concerned that these cases may be problematic. The histogram for the standardized residuals looks appropriate.

In the table above (Table 7.4), the studentized deleted residual is provided as a means of determining overly influential cases in our data set. Those cases exceeding a standardized value of 2.56 ($p < 0.01$) are cases with undue influence. Here, two cases (#28 and #57) exceed the 2.56 cutoff, and should be further evaluated. Note the case number is not the subject number in the data set, but literally the "row" number associated with the case.

The adjusted predicted value may also be evaluated for outliers by plotting it by the predicted value. Figure 7.5 presents the syntax and resulting plot. Cases that fall off the diagonal are indicative of possible outlying cases. In Figure 7.5, it appears most cases are in alignment.

The deleted residuals and studentized deleted residuals may also be evaluated for outliers. This is done by plotting the deleted residual by the calculated residual, and

Table 7.4 Outlier statistics, reprint courtesy of International Business Machines Corporation

Outlier Statistics[a]

		Case number	Statistics
Stud. Deleted Residual	1	28	3.346
	2	57	2.644
	3	73	−2.478
	4	55	2.172
	5	18	−2.089
	6	48	1.929
	7	12	1.616
	8	16	1.607
	9	35	1.590
	10	7	1.566

Source: © International Business Machines Corporation.

Note
a Dependent Variable: Vo$_2$mx_ml.

plotting the studentized deleted residual by the studentized residual. Cases that fall away from the diagonal are indicative of possible outlying cases. For both graphs (Figure 7.6), there is no evidence of outlying cases.

Influential data points

Influential data points may be examined using a centered leverage measure and Cook's distance (Cook's D). As shown in Table 7.5, we request a case-wise plot of

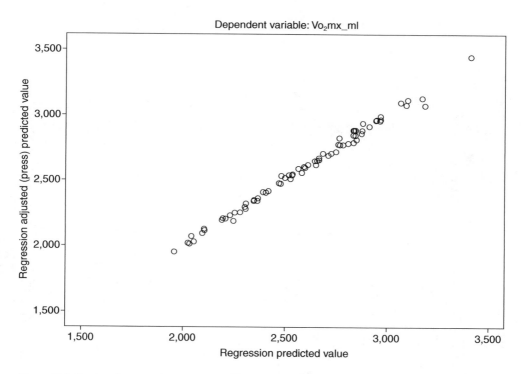

Figure 7.5 Scatterplot, reprint courtesy of International Business Machines Corporation.

Source: © International Business Machines Corporation.

Table 7.5 Casewise diagnostics, reprint courtesy of International Business Machines Corporation

Case number	Std. residual	Vo_2mx_ml	Residual	Centered leverage value	Cook's distance
28	2.947	4073	888.672	.096	.200
55	2.080	2934	627.136	.020	.026
57	2.468	3578	744.055	.040	.061
73	−2.287	2074	−689.569	.072	.088

Source: © International Business Machines Corporation.

Note
a Dependent Variable: Vo_2mx_ml.

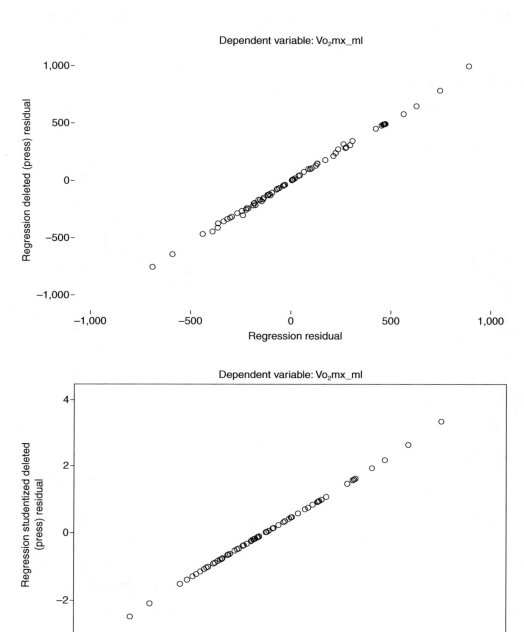

Figure 7.6 Scatterplot, reprint courtesy of International Business Machines Corporation.
Source: © International Business Machines Corporation.

cases with residuals greater than 2 using the "OUTLIERS(2)" command, which selects only those cases with standardized residuals ± 2. The residual (RESID) and standardized residual (ZRESID) is also presented for comparison purposes.

Using Formula 10.1 from earlier in the chapter, we calculate a leverage cutoff of 0.16. Below, k is the number of predictors in the regression, and N is the number of total cases. The values for leverage in Table 7.5 are all below the calculated cutoff of 0.16.

Leverage cutoff calculation

$$2\left(\frac{k+1}{N}\right) \tag{1}$$

$$2\left(\frac{5+1}{N}\right) \tag{2}$$

$$2\left(\frac{6}{75}\right) = 0.16 \tag{2}$$

For Cook's distance, we calculate a cutoff using $4/(N-2)$, with N being the total number of cases. For our example, we calculate a cutoff of 0.0548: $4/73 = 0.0548$. Next, we evaluate the extreme cases in the case-wise table from Table 7.5 – three of our cases violate the cutoff, and therefore may have an undue influence on the overall regression results.

Sample write-up

Typically, there is no write-up for the diagnostics analyses. These are performed prior to the formal regression analyses. Nevertheless, it is important to conduct these diagnostics as discussed above.

Using SPSS pulldown menu to generate histogram graph

1. Click **Graphs,** then move cursor over **Legacy Dialogs,** then over cursor over **Histogram** then left click.
2. Click **age_yrs,** then move to **Variable** box.
3. Then click **OK.**
4. Follow steps 1–3 to generate histogram for the oxygen uptake (Vo$_2$mx_ml) variable.

Syntax to generate histogram graph

GRAPH
/HISTOGRAM = age_yrs.
GRAPH
/HISTOGRAM = Vo$_2$mx_ml.

Using SPSS pulldown menu to generate bivariate scatter plot

1. Click **Graphs**, then move cursor over **Legacy Dialogs**, then over cursor over **Scatter/Dot** then left click.
2. Click **Simple Scatter** and then click **Define**.
3. Click **age_yrs** and move to X-axis box.
4. Click **Vo₂mx_ml** and move to Y-axis box.
5. Click **OK**.
6. Follow steps 1–5 to generate bivariate scatterplot for weight and oxygen uptake.

Syntax to generate bivariate scatterplots

GRAPH
/SCATTERPLOT(BIVAR)=age_yrs WITH Vo₂mx_ml
/MISSING=LISTWISE.
GRAPH
/SCATTERPLOT(BIVAR)=wt_kg WITH Vo₂mx_ml
/MISSING=LISTWISE.

Using SPSS pulldown menu for multivariate normality, linearity, and homoscedasticity

1. Click **Analyze**, then move cursor over **Regression** and then move cursor over **Linear** and click.
2. Click **Vo₂max_ml**, then move to Dependent box.
3. Click **wt_kg**, then move to Independent(s) box.
4. Click **ht_meter**, then move to Independent(s) box.
5. Click **age_yrs**, then move to Independent(s) box.
6. Click **Next**.
7. Click **timeperw**, then move to Independent(s) box.
8. Click **intensity**, then move to Independent(s) box.
9. You should now be on Block 2 of 2.
10. Click **Plots**, then click *****ZPRED**, and move to "X:" box.
11. Click **Plots**, then click *****ZRESID**, and move to "Y:" box.
12. Click **Continue**.
13. Click **OK**.

Syntax to generate multivariate normality, linearity, and homoscedasticity

REGRESSION
/MISSING LISTWISE
/STATISTICS COEFF OUTS R ANOVA
/CRITERIA=PIN(.05) POUT(.10) CIN(95)
/NOORIGIN
/DEPENDENT Vo₂mx_ml
/METHOD=ENTER wt_kg ht_meter age_yrs
/METHOD=ENTER timeperw intensty
/SCATTERPLOT=(*zresid,*zpred).

Using SPSS pulldown menu for bivariate correlations

1. Click **Analyze,** then move cursor over **Correlate** and then move cursor over **Bivariate** and click.
2. Click **Vo₂mx_ml,** then move to Variables box.
3. Repeat step #2 for wt_kg, ht_meter, age_yrs, timeperw, and intensity.
4. Note that Pearson is checked and two-tailed is also checked.
5. Flag significant correlations box should be checked.
6. Click **OK.**

Syntax to generate bivariate correlations

CORRELATION
/VARIABLES Vo₂mx_ml wt_kg ht_meter age_yrs timeperw intensty.

Using SPSS pulldown menu for tolerance and VIF

1. Click **Analyze,** then move cursor over **Regression** and then move cursor over **Linear** and click.
2. Click **Vo₂max_ml,** then move to Dependent box.
3. Click **wt_kg,** then move to Independent(s) box.
4. Click **ht_meter,** then move to Independent(s) box.
5. Click **age_yrs,** then move to Independent(s) box.
6. Click **Next.**
7. Click **timeperw,** then move to Independent(s) box.
8. Click **intensity,** then move to Independent(s) box.
9. You should now be on Block 2 of 2.
10. Click **Statistics,** then check the box for the following:

   a. Collinearity diagnostics.
   b. Confidence intervals level (%): 95.

11. Click **Continue.**
12. Click **OK.**

Syntax to generate tolerance and VIF

REGRESSION
/MISSING LISTWISE
/STATISTICS COEFF OUTS CI(95) R ANOVA COLLIN TOL
/CRITERIA=PIN(.05) POUT(.10)
/NOORIGIN
/DEPENDENT Vo₂mx_ml
/METHOD=ENTER wt_kg ht_meter age_yrs
/METHOD=ENTER timeperw intensty.

Using SPSS Pulldown Menu for Independence of Errors (Durbin-Watson Test)

1. Click **Analyze,** then move cursor over **Regression** and then move cursor over **Linear** and click.

2. Click **Vo₂max_ml,** then move to Dependent box.
3. Click **wt_kg,** then move to Independent(s) box.
4. Click **ht_meter,** then move to Independent(s) box.
5. Click **age_yrs,** then move to Independent(s) box.
6. Click **Next.**
7. Click **timeperw,** then move to Independent(s) box.
8. Click **intensity,** then move to Independent(s) box.
9. You should now be on Block 2 of 2.
10. Click **Statistics,** then check the box for the following:

    a.   Collinearity diagnostics.
    b.   Confidence intervals level (%): 95.
    c.   Durbin-Watson.

11. Click **Continue.**
12. Click **OK.**

Syntax to generate independence of errors (Durbin-Watson test)

REGRESSION
/MISSING LISTWISE
/STATISTICS COEFF OUTS CI(95) R ANOVA
/CRITERIA=PIN(.05) POUT(.10)
/NOORIGIN
/DEPENDENT Vo₂mx_ml
/METHOD=ENTER wt_kg ht_meter age_yrs
/METHOD=ENTER timeperw intensty
/RESIDUALS DURBIN.

Using SPSS pulldown menu standardized residuals

1. Click **Analyze,** then move cursor over **Regression** and then move cursor over **Linear** and click.
2. Click **Vo₂max_ml,** then move to Dependent box.
3. Click **wt_kg,** then move to Independent(s) box.
4. Click **ht_meter,** then move to Independent(s) box.
5. Click **age_yrs,** then move to Independent(s) box.
6. Click **Next.**
7. Click **timeperw,** then move to Independent(s) box.
8. Click **intensity,** then move to Independent(s) box.
9. You should now be on Block 2 of 2.
10. Click **Paste.**

    a.   This will bring up the syntax window with your syntax for the above steps.
    b.   Then type in the following syntax on the last line:

        i.   /residuals=histogram(sdresid) outliers(sdresid).

11. Then click the green play (▶) icon on the top of the menu.

Syntax to generate standardized residuals

REGRESSION
/MISSING LISTWISE
/STATISTICS COEFF OUTS R ANOVA
/CRITERIA=PIN(.05) POUT(.10) CIN(95)
/NOORIGIN
/DEPENDENT Vo_2mx_ml
/METHOD=ENTER wt_kg ht_meter age_yrs
/METHOD=ENTER timeperw intensty
/residuals=histogram(sdresid) outliers(sdresid).

Using SPSS pulldown menu for adjusted predicted values

1. Click **Analyze**, then move cursor over **Regression** and then move cursor over **Linear** and click.
2. Click **Vo_2max_ml**, then move to Dependent box.
3. Click **wt_kg**, then move to Independent(s) box.
4. Click **ht_meter**, then move to Independent(s) box.
5. Click **age_yrs**, then move to Independent(s) box.
6. Click **Next**.
7. Click **timeperw**, then move to Independent(s) box.
8. Click **intensity**, then move to Independent(s) box.
9. You should now be on Block 2 of 2.
10. Click **Paste**.

    a.   This will bring up the syntax window with your syntax for the above steps.
    b.   Then type in the following syntax on the last line:

         i.   /SCATTERPLOT=(*adjpred, *pred).

11. Then click the green play (▶) icon on the top of the menu.

Syntax to generate adjusted predicted values

REGRESSION
/MISSING LISTWISE
/STATISTICS COEFF OUTS R ANOVA
/CRITERIA=PIN(.05) POUT(.10) CIN(95)
/NOORIGIN
/DEPENDENT Vo_2mx_ml
/METHOD=ENTER wt_kg ht_meter age_yrs
/METHOD=ENTER timeperw intensty
/SCATTERPLOT=(*adjpred, *pred).

Using SPSS pulldown menu for deleted residuals and studentized deleted residuals

1. Click **Analyze**, then move cursor over **Regression** and then move cursor over **Linear** and click.

2. Click **Vo₂max_ml,** then move to Dependent box.
3. Click **wt_kg,** then move to Independent(s) box.
4. Click **ht_meter,** then move to Independent(s) box.
5. Click **age_yrs,** then move to Independent(s) box.
6. Click **Next.**
7. Click **timeperw,** then move to Independent(s) box.
8. Click **intensity,** then move to Independent(s) box.
9. You should now be on Block 2 of 2.
10. Click **Paste.**

    a.   This will bring up the syntax window with your syntax for the above steps.

    b.   Then type in the following syntax on the last line:

         i.   /SCATTERPLOT=(*DRESID, *RESID) (*SDRESID, *SRESID).

11. Then click the green play (▶) icon on the top of the menu.

Syntax to generate deleted residuals and studentized deleted residuals

REGRESSION
/MISSING LISTWISE
/STATISTICS COEFF OUTS R ANOVA
/CRITERIA=PIN(.05) POUT(.10) CIN(95)
/NOORIGIN
/DEPENDENT Vo₂mx_ml
/METHOD=ENTER wt_kg ht_meter age_yrs
/METHOD=ENTER timeperw intensty
/SCATTERPLOT=(*DRESID, *RESID) (*SDRESID, *SRESID).

Using SPSS pulldown menu for leverage and Cook's D

1. Click **Analyze,** then move cursor over **Regression** and then move cursor over **Linear** and click.
2. Click **Vo₂max_ml,** then move to Dependent box.
3. Click **wt_kg,** then move to Independent(s) box.
4. Click **ht_meter,** then move to Independent(s) box.
5. Click **age_yrs,** then move to Independent(s) box.
6. Click **Next.**
7. Click **timeperw,** then move to Independent(s) box.
8. Click **intensity,** then move to Independent(s) box.
9. You should now be on Block 2 of 2.
10. Click **Paste.**

    a.   This will bring up the syntax window with your syntax for the above steps.

    b.   Then type in the following syntax on the last line:

         i.   /casewise=resid zresid cook lever outliers(2).

11. Then click the green play (▶) icon on the top of the menu.

Syntax to generate for leverage and Cook's D

REGRESSION
/MISSING LISTWISE
/STATISTICS COEFF OUTS R ANOVA
/CRITERIA=PIN(.05) POUT(.10) CIN(95)
/NOORIGIN
/DEPENDENT Vo_2mx_ml
/METHOD=ENTER wt_kg ht_meter age_yrs
/METHOD=ENTER timeperw intensty
/casewise=resid zresid cook lever outliers(2).

8 Basic multiple regression analysis

Introduction

Multiple regression is a statistical technique designed to assess the association between multiple variables and the outcome variable. For example, the investigator may be interested in examining the relationship between upper body strength and distance the javelin is thrown, $\dot{V}o_2$ max and 1.5 mile run time, or grade point average and hours spent studying. Regression may be conceived as an extension of correlation, with the goal being prediction of an outcome from a set of predictor variables. The predictor variables may be viewed as independent variables, and the outcome variable is a dependent variable. One advantage of using regression over correlation is the technique allows the overlaps or correlations across predictor variables to be taken into account when predicting an outcome.

The investigator can use multiple regression for a number of aims. For example, multiple regression is used to assess the overall association of a set of predictors on an outcome. Another aim is to derive a model of prediction, which may be used if the investigator wishes to predict an outcome from a set of predictor variables. A third aim is to assess the importance of predictors. Lastly, multiple regression can be used to explore various predictors and their associations with an outcome.

Research questions

What is the overall association between a set of predictors and an outcome? Multiple regression allows for an examination of the association between a set of predictors and an outcome. Regression produces a multiple R test statistic to indicate the overall association between a set of predictors and a criterion, and whether this multiple correlation is different than what would be expected by chance occurrence.

An overall model of prediction can be derived using the resulting multiple regression parameters to derive a model: $Y' = a + b_1x_1 + b_2x_2 + \ldots + b_ix_i$. Here, Y' is the predicted score for the outcome variable. The b values are regression parameters, also known as weights, derived through multiple regression. The x values are data values from the predictor variables. This formula may be used to predict future scores on the outcome variable. For example, you may be interested in predicting force production (i.e., torque) as a function of age. The resulting model can also be assessed as to its significance and whether there is a linear association between the set of predictor variables and a criterion.

Which are the most important predictor variables? Multiple regression can be used to assess the most important predictor variables from a set. Because of preexisting correlations between predictor variables, correlations alone may be inaccurate to assess the importance of variables in their association with an outcome since independent variables will typically overlap. Taking into account the overlap across predictors, multiple regression can be used to evaluate the most important predictors in a model. In addition, the technique can assess whether each variable contributes uniquely to the overall regression results. Another question addressed through multiple regression includes comparing sets of predictor variables – is one set of predictor variables superior to another set?

A host of exploratory data analysis techniques are also available in multiple regression. These techniques, referred to as exploratory statistical approaches, allow for specific statistical criterion to be utilized in the selection of predictors. Three statistical approaches to exploratory regression, called Forward, Backward, and Stepwise, are commonly used. We **discourage** the use of these exploratory regression techniques to develop the prediction model because they often capitalize on chance. Instead, however, we recommend that investigators use hierarchical linear regression (2) for model building. Hierarchical linear regression is preferable, because the investigator controls the order of entry of predictor variables based on theoretical considerations as well as less capitalization on chance (1). Alternatively, we also recommend the use of the standard multiple regression approach, where all predictor variables are entered simultaneously into the model for evaluation. The one limitation, however, with this approach is that the investigators will not be able to determine if a set of predictors improves the overall regression model above and beyond another set of predictors.

Review of regression analysis

Multiple regression is based on the statistical method *ordinary least squares* (OLS), which allows for the best linear fit of predictors to an outcome. A simple general linear model may be used for illustration. The following example pertains to two variables; one predictor (X) and one outcome (Y):

$$Y' = A + BX$$

Formula 8.1

Predicted criterion Y'. Y' is the predicted outcome. It is the resulting predicted value which corresponds to the derived linear fit of a subject's score X on the predictor variable Y.

Regression weight "B." B is the *regression weight*, and is used to multiply each subject's score on the predictor variable. It is also referred to as the *slope* to indicate the direction of the regression line (e.g., a positive slope $\angle$ or negative slope $\searrow$).

The formula for slope B is as follows:

$$B = \frac{\sum (X - \bar{X})(Y - \bar{Y})}{\sum (X - \bar{X})^2}$$

Formula 8.2

In formula 8.2, the numerator is a measure of *covariance*, which is an indicator of how much variables move together. For both X and Y, mean deviations are calculated and multiplied together and summed. Larger mean deviations will yield a greater covariance. Note that the numerator for B is exactly the same as the numerator for the Pearson correlation coefficient. Once the covariance is known, it is divided by the sum of squares for X. Mean deviations are taken for X, squared, and summed. The resulting slope is an indicator of the regression line's trajectory. If the slope is zero, then the expected association between X and Y would be flat, $\vert\!\!-\!\!-$. A positive slope indicates a positive association, $\vert\!\diagup$, while a negative slope represents a declining association, $\vert\diagdown$.

Intercept "A." A is the <u>intercept</u>, and is a constant added to each subject's score on the predictor variable. The formula for the intercept A is as follows:

$$A = \bar{Y} - B\bar{X} \qquad \text{Formula 8.3}$$

For formula 8.3, the mean value for Y is subtracted from the product of slope and the mean of X.

Forming the regression line. The slope B and intercept A are used to represent the straight-line association or line of best fit between the X and Y variables. If a scatterplot of X and Y are produced, the value for A is the point where the regression line starts on the Y axis of the scatterplot. The value of B is the gradient or slope of the regression line. It also represents how Y changes with unit increases in X.

Values for A and B in the model are derived to minimize the difference between the predicted outcome Y' and the actual value. The difference between Y' and Y is the <u>residual</u>: $Y' - Y = Residual$. Therefore, values of A and B that provide the smallest set of residuals are chosen as the final values in the general linear regression model.

Sum of squares for Y and ANOVA. In addition to the OLS equation, an assessment of the overall linear model is made by calculating the total sum of squares on Y (representing variability in Y). This is partitioned into a component reflecting variance associated with the regression line, and an error variance component reflecting deviations of scores from the regression line.

$$SS_y = SS_{reg} + SS_{res} \qquad \text{Formula 8.4}$$

$$SS_y = \sum(Y - \bar{Y})^2 \qquad (1)$$

$$SS_{reg} = \sum(Y' - \bar{Y})^2 \qquad (2)$$

$$SS_{res} = \sum(Y - Y')^2 \qquad (3)$$

The sum of squares values SS_{reg} and SS_{res} can be converted in the typical format to mean square estimates by dividing by the appropriate degrees of freedom values (1 and N-2), and an F-ratio may be derived to assess the significance of the linear model.

Multiple R-square. A multiple R-square value r_{xy}^2, also known as the <u>coefficient of determination</u>, may be calculated using the SS_y and SS_{reg} components. Multiple R-square is a measure of the percent variance accounted for in the criterion Y by the predictor X, and also a measure of the relationship strength between the variables. By taking the square root of R-square, a multiple R is produced.

$$r_{xy}^2 = \frac{SS_{reg}}{SS_y} \qquad \text{Formula 8.5}$$

Adjusted R-square. The adjusted R-square value r^2_{adj} adjusts the sample r-square value so it is a better estimate of the underlying association in the population.

$$r^2_{adj} = r^2_{xy} - \frac{p(1 - r^2_{xy})}{N - p - 1}$$

Formula 8.6

Here, N is the total number of participants in the sample, and p is the total number of predictor variables.

Standard error of the regression weight, standardized weight, and significance test. Earlier, the formula for the regression weight was presented. The standard error of this weight may also be calculated to provide the standard deviation of the weight in the general population. This is done by first calculating the standard error of the estimate of Y:

$$s_{y.x} = s_y \sqrt{1 - r^2_{xy}}$$

Formula 8.7

Where s_y is the standard deviation of the criterion Y. Knowing the standard error of the estimate, the standard error of B can now be taken

$$se_B = \frac{s_{y.x}}{\sqrt{\sum x^2}}$$

Formula 8.8

Where the standard error of the estimate $s_{y.x}$ is divided by the square root of the sum of the predictor squared.

The significance of the regression coefficient may be tested using a t-test distribution with the following formula and a degrees of freedom of $N-2$:

$$t_B = \frac{B}{SE_B}$$

Formula 8.9

The regression weight may also be standardized to allow for direct comparisons across multiple predictors. When the regression weight is standardized, the standardized coefficient is called *Beta*.

$$\beta = B\left(\frac{S_x}{S_y}\right)$$

Formula 8.10

Here, β is a function of the regression weight multiplied by the ratio between the standard deviations of X and Y.

Limitations of multiple regression

The resulting associations between the predictors and the outcome are not causal unless the research was designed for such purposes. If the predictors are true independent variables which were manipulated to effect an outcome, then causality can be concluded. In the majority of applications of multiple regression, however, data are used to investigate associations and prediction, not causation.

Another limitation is that data used for multiple regression should be continuous, although two-level discrete or dichotomous data may be used as predictors. *Note that if the outcome variable or dependent variable is dichotomous, multiple regression is the wrong technique. Instead, use logistic regression, which allows for dichotomous or categorical outcomes.* If predictor variables are discrete with more than two levels, you may still use the data in multiple regression, but data should be coded in a specific format called <u>dummy coding</u>. The resulting multiple regression model is solely limited to the variables used in the analysis. If variables were poorly envisioned or measured, then it is doubtful the research will be reliable.

Example of multiple regression (example 1)

Do indices of habitual physical activity contribute to the prediction of $\dot{V}o_2$ max in aerobically trained women above and beyond traditional predictors such as body weight, height, and age?

Using SPSS pulldown menu for hierarchical regression (example 1)

1. Click **Analyze,** then click **Regression,** then click **Linear.**
2. Click **wt_kg** and move to Independent(s) box.
3. Click **ht_meter** and move to Independent(s) box.
4. Click **age_yrs** and move to Independent(s) box, then click **Next.**
5. Click **timeperw** and move to Independent(s) box.
6. Click **intensity** and move to Independent(s) box.

   a.   At this point you should be on block 2 of 2.

7. Click **Vo₂max_ml** and move to Dependent box.
8. Click **Statistics.**

   a.   Estimates and Model Fit should already be checked off.
   b.   You need to click the box for R-squared change.
   c.   You need to click the box for Descriptives.
   d.   Click **Continue.**

9. Click **OK.**

Syntax for SPSS for hierarchical regression (example 1)

```
REGRESSION
/DESCRIPTIVES MEAN STDDEV CORR SIG N
/MISSING LISTWISE
/STATISTICS COEFF OUTS R ANOVA CHANGE
/CRITERIA=PIN(.05) POUT(.10)
/NOORIGIN
/DEPENDENT Vo₂mx_ml
/METHOD=ENTER wt_kg ht_meter age_yrs
/METHOD=ENTER timeperw intensty.
```

Interpreting the output for hierarchical regression (example 1)

The IBM SPSS Statistics software (SPSS) output begins with basic descriptive information on the variables used for the regression. Basic descriptive statistics are produced by the "Descriptives" command in the syntax, and include the mean, standard deviation, and available N (nonmissing) for each variable. Note also that in the SPSS syntax, a "Missing Listwise" command was used, which is the default setting in SPSS. Only those cases with complete data on all variables are utilized in the analysis. Since multiple regression analyses are based on the resulting correlation matrix among variables, listwise deletion is our recommendation since all of the correlations are based on the same N. An alternative would be "Missing Pairwise" which we do not recommend. If the "Pairwise" command is used, the resulting correlation matrix would be based on differing pairwise N combinations, which can introduce bias into the analyses.

Following "Descriptives" is information on the entry of variables under the heading "Variables Entered/Removed." For Model 1, age, weight, and height are slated for simultaneous entry into the regression equation. Model 2 will add times per week subjects exercised, and intensity of training into the model.

The next portion of output, entitled "Model Summary," provides information for each model step. The statistics provided include multiple R, multiple R-square, the adjusted multiple R-square, and a test of R-square change. Results for the Model 1 predictors (age, weight, and height) show that the **multiple R** is 0.65. The **multiple**

Table 8.1 Descriptive statistics, reprint courtesy of International Business Machines Corporation

Descriptive Statistics

	Mean	Std. deviation	N
Vo$_2$mx_ml	2589.15	435.24	75
wt_kg	60.53	7.97	75
ht_meter	1.66	.07	75
age_yrs	38.24	9.56	75
Times/wk_exercise	6.72	2.37	75
Intensity of subjects training (6–20)	13.65	1.68	75

Source: © International Business Machines Corporation.

Table 8.2 Variables entered/removed, reprint courtesy of International Business Machines Corporation

Variables Entered/Removed[a]

Model	Variables entered	Variables removed	Method
1	age_yrs, wt_kg, ht_meter[b]		Enter
2	Times/wk_exercise, intensity of subjects training (6–20)[b]		Enter

Source: © International Business Machines Corporation.

Notes
a Dependent Variable: Vo$_2$mx_ml.
b All requested variables entered.

R-square is 0.42, indicating that 42 percent of the total variation in volume of oxygen is accounted for by these three variables. The **adjusted R-square** is 0.40, which is an adjustment for R-square for generalization to a broader population. The **R-square change** is the change in R-square from the previous model to the current model. Here, the previous model (not shown) is the null model containing no predictors, and thus generating an R-square value of 0. Model 1 has an R-square value of 0.42. Therefore, the R-square change value is 0.42: $0.42_{Model1} - 0_{Null\ Model} = 0.42$. This change of 0.42 is then assessed using ANOVA (F_{Change}) to evaluate whether the R-square change value of 0.42 is above and beyond what would be expected by chance occurrence. For Model 1, the R-square change of 0.42 is significant, $F(3, 71) = 17.30$, $p < 0.001$, suggesting that the resulting R-square change (from the null model) is unlikely to have occurred by chance.

Model 2 is evaluated the same way (Table 8.3). Two additional variables are added to the model – times per week exercising, and intensity of training. With five total variables in the model, the **multiple R** is 0.74. The **multiple R-square** is 0.55, indicating 55 percent of the total variation in volume of oxygen is accounted for by the five predictors. The **adjusted R-square** is 0.52, and reflects the change in R-square from Model 1 to Model 2. The Model 1 R-square was 0.42, and the Model 2 R-square was 0.55. Thus, the R-square change value is 0.13: $0.55_{Model\ 2} - 0.42_{Model\ 1} = 0.13$. This change of 0.13 from Model 1 to Model 2 indicates that times per week exercising and intensity of training, when added to the regression model, account for an additional 13 percent of the variance in volume of oxygen. In other words, above and beyond the variables in Model 1, the addition of these two variables accounts for an additional 13 percent of the variance in our criterion. An ANOVA F_{Change} is next provided to evaluate whether the R-square change value of 0.13 is beyond what would be expected by chance occurrence. For Model 2, the R-square change of 0.13 is significant, $F(2, 69) = 10.04$, $p < 0.001$, suggesting that the resulting increase in R-square by the addition of the two new variables is unlikely to have occurred by chance.

Next in the SPSS output are the assessments of the overall linear model for the variables in each model, under the heading "ANOVA." For Model 1 with the three predictors in the model, a significant F statistic is noted, $F(3, 71) = 17.30$, $p < 0.001$. This ANOVA tells us that there is a significant linear association between the three predictors in Model 1 and the criterion. For Model 2, with all five predictors in the model, there is a significant F statistic, $F(5, 69) = 17.04$, $p < 0.001$. Again, this indicates a significant linear association between the five predictors and the criterion.

Table 8.3 Model summary, reprint courtesy of International Business Machines Corporation
Model Summary

Model	R	R-square	Adjusted R-square	Std. error of the estimate
1	.650[a]	.422	.398	337.741
2	.743[b]	.553	.520	301.511

Source: © International Business Machines Corporation.

Notes
a Predictors: (Constant), age_yrs, wt_kg, ht_meter.
b Predictors: (Constant), age_yrs, wt_kg, ht_meter, Times/wk_exercise, intensity of subjects training (6–20).

Table 8.4 ANOVA, reprint courtesy of International Business Machines Corporation
ANOVA[a]

Model		Sum of squares	df.	Mean square	F	Sig.
1	Regression	5919109.089	3	1973036.363	17.297	.000[b]
	Residual	8098878.298	71	114068.708		
	Total	14017987.39	74			
2	Regression	7745277.629	5	1549055.526	17.040	.000[c]
	Residual	6272709.758	69	90908.837		
	Total	14017987.39	74			

Source: © International Business Machines Corporation.

Notes
a Dependent Variable: Vo_2mx_ml
b Predictors: (Constant), age_yrs, wt_kg, ht_meter.
c Predictors: (Constant), age_yrs, wt_kg, ht_meter, Times/wk_exercise, intensity of subjects training (6–20).

The last portion of output entitled "Coefficients" concerns the components of the OLS regression equation. Under the column "Unstandardized Coefficients" is the **regression weight or slope B**, followed by the **standard error of the regression weight** SE_β. The next main column heading is "Standardized Coefficients" and contains the **standardized regression weights** (β's). The final two columns contain the **significance test (using a *t*-test) of the regression weights**. The **intercept A** is located in the row marked as "(Constant)."

Looking at the "Unstandardized Coefficients" column for Model 1, the OLS regression equation components can easily be identified. The intercept is –1422.79 (listed as

Table 8.5 Coefficients, reprint courtesy of International Business Machines Corporation
Coefficients[a]

Model		Unstandardized coefficients		Standardized coefficients	t	Sig.
		B	Std. error	Beta		
1	(Constant)	–1422.789	1183.064		–1.303	.233
	wt_kg	9.443	6.260	.173	1.508	.136
	ht_meter	2403.429	785.990	.371	3.058	.003
	age_yrs	–14.082	4.433	–.309	–3.177	.002
2	(Constant)	–2236.488	1072.522		–2.085	.041
	wt_kg	16.462	5.824	.302	2.827	.006
	ht_meter	1785.958	715.362	.276	2.497	.015
	age_yrs	–12.601	3.980	–.277	–3.166	.002
	Times/wk_exercise	7.704	15.281	.042	.504	.616
	Intensity of subjects training (6–20)	95.407	22.354	.368	4.268	.000

Source: © International Business Machines Corporation.

Note
a Dependent Variable: Vo_2mx_ml

"constant"), and the regression weights are 9.44 for weight, 2403.43 for height, and −14.08 for age. Together, the regression equation would be:

$$\dot{V}o_2 \max = -1422.79 + 9.44(\text{weight}) + 2403.43(\text{height}) + -14.08(\text{age})$$

The most important predictors in Model 1 may be ascertained by evaluating the standardized regression weights (ß's). The variable with the largest ß-value is height (0.37), followed by age (−0.31) and weight (0.17). The significance of the predictors is next evaluated, which shows only two of the predictors, height and age, are significant at $p \leq 0.05$. Although the intercept A is also provided a t-test, this test is evaluated only in specific circumstances. Here, it will be disregarded.

Model 2 is interpreted in a similar fashion. The intercept for Model 2 is −2236.49, and the regression weights are 16.46 for weight, 1785.96 for height, −12.60 for age, 7.70 for times per week exercising, and 95.41 for intensity of training. Together, the regression equation would be:

$$\dot{V}o_2 \max = -2236.49 + 16.46(\text{weight}) + 1785.96(\text{height}) + -12.60(\text{age}) + 7.70$$
(exercise per week) + 95.41(training intensity)

Which are the most important predictors in Model 2? The variable with the largest ß is intensity of training (0.37), followed by weight (0.30) and age (−0.28). The significance of the predictors is next evaluated, which shows four of the five predictors being significant at $p \leq 0.05$. The one nonsignificant predictor is times per week exercising.

Sample write-up for hierarchical regression (example 1)

In the present study, hierarchical linear regression was used to determine predictors of $\dot{V}o_2$ *max*. We first entered anthropometric measures into the first block and found a significant increase in the R-value (R = 0.65; $p < 0.001$). In the second block we entered measurement related to exercise intensity. As a result, we found that the R-value significantly increased (R = 0.74; $p < 0.001$). Therefore, the total variance accounted for by the model was 52 percent ($R^2 = 0.52$) using the following equation: 16.462(wt_kg) + 1785.958(ht_meter) − 12.601(age_yrs) + 7.704(times/wk_exercise) + 95.407 (intensity of subjects training) − 2236.488.

Example of multiple regression (example 2)

In this second example, rather than performing a hierarchical linear regression the investigator is interested in placing all the predictors into a single block and then determining which predictors are significantly contributing to the model. To keep this example simplistic, there are four predictor variables and then the dependent variable.

Using SPSS pulldown menu for a single block regression (example 2)

1. Click **Analyze**, then click **Regression**, then click **Linear**.

2. *Hold down the CTRL key*, and then click **predictor_1, predictor_2, predictor_3, predictor_4**, and move to Independent(s) box.
3. Click **dependent_variable** and move to the Dependent box.
4. At this point, all the predictors are in Block 1 of 1.
5. Click **Statistics**.

    a. Estimates and Model Fit should already be checked off.
    b. You need to click the box for R-squared change.
    c. You need to click the box for Descriptives.
    d. Click **Continue**.

6. Click **OK**.

Syntax for SPSS for a single block regression (example 2)

```
REGRESSION
/DESCRIPTIVES MEAN STDDEV CORR SIG N
/MISSING LISTWISE
/STATISTICS COEFF OUTS R ANOVA CHANGE
/CRITERIA=PIN(.05) POUT(.10)
/NOORIGIN
/DEPENDENT Dependent_variable
/METHOD=ENTER Predictor_1 Predictor_2 Predictor_3 Predictor_4.
```

Interpreting the output for a single block regression (example 2)

As shown in Table 8.6, the model summary indicates that for this single block, the R-square change value (0.517) is statistically significant from zero as indicated in the column labeled "Sig. F Change." Thus, the R-value for this model is $R = 0.719$ and the SEE is 0.794.

Table 8.7 is the ANOVA table and show a significant F statistic [$F_{(4, 233)} = 58.510$; $p < 0.001$]. This ANOVA table tells us that there is a significant linear association between the four predictors in Model 1 and the criterion (i.e., dependent variable).

The "Coefficients" is shown in Table 8.8 which provide information regarding the regression weight, standard error of the regression weight, standardized

Table 8.6 Model summary, reprint courtesy of International Business Machines Corporation
Model Summary

Model	R	R-square	Adjusted R-square	Std. error of the estimate	Change statistics				
					R-square change	F change	df1	df2	Sig. F change
1	.719[a]	.517	.508	.79416	.517	58.510	4	219	.000

Source: © International Business Machines Corporation.

Note
a Predictors: (Constant), Predictor_4, Predictor_2, Predictor_1, Predictor_3.

regression weights, and the significance test of the regression weights. We can see that predictors 3 and 4 significantly contribute to the model, whereas predictors 1 and 2 do not (*p*-values 0.101 and 0.275, respectively). In addition, an examination of the standardized regression weights (β) predictor 3 had the largest value ($\beta = 0.567$) compared to predictor 3 ($\beta = 0.289$).

Sample write-up for the single block regression (example 2)

In the current study, we investigated whether or not four variables were good predictors for our outcome variable. Therefore, we entered all four predictors into a single block with our outcome variable as the dependent variable. The linear regression revealed a significant increase in R-value (R = 0.719, SEE = 0.794; $p < 0.001$). We found that predictors 3 and 4 significantly contributed to the model, but not predictors 1 and 2. Moreover, the β-weights show that predictor 3 uniquely contributed to the model ($\beta = 0.567$) than predictor 4 ($\beta = 0.289$). Thus, the total variance accounted for by the model was 52 percent ($R^2 = 0.517$) using the following equation: 0.339(predictor 3) + 0.077(predictor 4) + 2.275.

Table 8.7 ANOVA, reprint courtesy of International Business Machines Corporation
ANOVA[a]

Model		Sum of squares	df.	Mean square	F	Sig.
1	Regression	147.609	4	36.902	58.510	.000
	Residual	138.122	219	.631		
	Total	285.731	223			

Source: © International Business Machines Corporation.

Note
a Dependent Variable: Dependent_variable.

Table 8.8 Coefficients, reprint courtesy of International Business Machines Corporation
Coefficients[a]

Model		Unstandardized coefficients		Standardized coefficients	t	Sig.
		B	Std. error	Beta		
1	(Constant)	2.275	.382		5.949	.000
	Predictor_1	.199	.121	.081	1.647	.101
	Predictor_2	−.013	.012	−.052	−1.095	.275
	Predictor_3	.339	.030	.567	11.289	.000
2	Predictor_4	.077	.013	.289	5.968	.000

Source: © International Business Machines Corporation.

Note
a Dependent Variable: Dependent_variable.

References

1. Berger DE. Using regression analysis., in: *Handbook of practical program evaluation*. JS Wholey, HP Hatry, KE Newcomer, eds. San Francisco: John Wiley & Sons, 2004, pp. 479–505.
2. Malek MH, Berger DE, and Coburn JW. On the inappropriateness of stepwise regression analysis for model building and testing. *European Journal of Applied Physiology* 101: 263–264; author reply 265–266, 2007.

9 Multiple regression models for quantitative and categorical data

Introduction

As discussed in Chapter 8, multiple regression is a statistical tool used to determine the association of multiple variables on an outcome. In this chapter, we will provide examples of model building with quantitative and categorical data. Categorical data are variables that are mutually exclusive such as ethnicity, religion, or gender. For continuous variables participants may vary in terms of amount, whereas for categorical variables participants vary in type. It should be noted, however, that if appropriate a continuous variable can also be transformed into a categorical variable. For example, the investigator may be interested in examining age groups on a dependent variable (i.e., strength performance). In this case, the investigator has recorded the age of each subject, but wants to examine the association of age group on the dependent variable. Therefore, the investigator can create a categorical variable such as 20–29, 30–39, and 40–49 years old and then determine how many of the subjects fit into each category.

Curvilinear regression

In addition to examining quantitative and categorical data we will also introduce curvilinear regression model development. It should be noted that there are two approaches available for curvilinear analyses: powered vectors and orthogonal polynomials (16). For the purposes of this book we will focus on the more common powered vectors regression as it has been typically used in the exercise science literature. Polynomial regression models[1] are an extension of linear models (16).

Below is the transformation of the linear regression model to a powered vector regression model:

$$Y = b_0 + m_1 X \qquad \text{(Equation 1, Linear Model)}$$

$$Y = b_0 + m_1 X + m_2 X^2 \qquad \text{(Equation 2, Quadratic Model)}$$

$$Y = b_0 + m_1 X + m_2 X^2 + m_3 X^3 \qquad \text{(Equation 3, Cubic Model)}$$

where $m_2 X^2$ and $m_3 X^3$ are the squared and cubed slope terms for equations 2 and 3, respectively. Typically, the quadratic regression line has one bend, whereas the cubic regression line has two bends. To determine if one model is significantly different from another, the increment in the proportion of the variance accounted for by the higher-degree model or trend is determined by using an *F*-test assessing the R-square change. This will be shown in the SPSS output later in this chapter.

Regression with categorical variables

Categorical data require special treatment in multiple regression because data are required to be at least interval level for both the criterion and predictors, and most categorical or discrete data are nominal (the one exception is dichotomous data). As a general rule, if your *criterion variable* is nominal or dichotomous, multiple regression is the <u>wrong</u> technique. Instead, *logistic regression* is the appropriate technique to use when outcome measures are dichotomous or multinomial.

If the *predictor variables* are dichotomous, they may be used in multiple regression. However, if the predictor variables are multinomial, they must be altered for use in multiple regression. The coding technique used to alter multinomial variables in regression is *dummy coding*. For dummy coding, we create $k-1$ number of new variables to represent the categories of a multinomial variable, with k indicating the total number of categories. The new variables created are called *dummy variables*. Thus, if there five categories, 5–1 dummy variables would be created. The dummy variables consist of 0's and 1's, with "0" indicating no membership or representation in a category, and "1" indicating membership. The $k-1$ dummy variables are then used as a "variable set" to represent the multinomial variable in multiple regression.

To illustrate dummy coding, say the investigator has a multinomial variable indicating the race/ethnicity of people in the sample: White, Latino, African-American, and Mixed/Other race. We would create $k-1$ number of dummy variables – in this case, we might consider creating a dummy variable for White, one for Latino, and one for African-American. We do not need to create a dummy variable for Mixed/Other race since that category is implicit in the other dummy variables (if the subject is not White, or Latino, or African-American, they must be Mixed/Other race). The category that is not dummy coded is called the *reference group* (in our example, Mixed/Other race). For some regression applications, the category chosen as the reference group is not important. However, there are instances when choice of the reference group can provide pertinent information in the regression model.

To dummy code, the race/ethnicity variable, create the three dummy variables noted above. This is shown in Table 9.1 on a small sample of 10 cases. If someone is White, they are given a "1" for the White dummy variable. If they are not White, they are given a "0." We do the same for the Latino dummy variable, and for the African-American dummy variable. Notice that Mixed/Other race membership is represented by having all 0's in the three dummy variables.

Once the dummy variables have been created, they are used in hierarchical regression as a "set" to ascertain the unique contribution of the multinomial variable. In our working example, the three dummy variables would be entered together as a separate model in hierarchical regression to represent race/ethnicity.

Hierarchical versus statistical regression

In developing a regression model (or equation) it is imperative for the <u>investigator</u> and <u>not</u> the statistical program to determine the independent variables that make up

Table 9.1 Dummy coding example using race/ethnicity as the categorical variable

Subject	Race/ethnicity	Dummy variables		
		White	*Latino*	*African-American*
1	White	1	0	0
2	White	1	0	0
3	White	1	0	0
4	Latino	0	1	0
5	Latino	0	1	0
6	African-American	0	0	1
7	African-American	0	0	1
8	African-American	0	0	1
9	Mixed/Other	0	0	0
10	Mixed/Other	0	0	0

the prediction model. This approach is called "statistical regression" and, unfortunately, many investigators use this technique when generating their regression model. Statistical regression consists of three different analytic methods; *forward, backward*, and *stepwise*. Forward regression allows items into the regression equation sequentially based solely on an adopted statistical criterion (usually the significance of the partial correlation of a predictor with the criterion). Once items are in the model, they cannot be removed. Backward regression enters all items into the regression model, then removes items sequentially based on the assigned statistical criterion. The stepwise approach combines both the forward and backward approaches; items are sequentially entered into the regression model based on a statistical criterion, and in later models items are evaluated for removal using a different criterion. The key in all of these approaches is that variable inclusion and exclusion is driven solely by the statistical criterion adopted, and not by the researcher.

Statistical regression has a number of drawbacks, and therefore we cannot recommend the technique. First, the resulting model may be nonsensible, meaning that the final variables chosen based on the statistical criterion may not make theoretical sense. Second, the statistical criterion used to select variables may be too liberal, with too many variables included in the model. Third, the statistical criterion used to select variables may be too conservative, with too few variables included in the model. Fourth, researchers sometimes overemphasize the final model as being correct, when in fact it was generated solely on the basis of the statistic criterion and the sample data. If another sample were drawn from the same population, there is a good chance that statistical regression would generate different results. Fifth, for some forms of statistical regression (i.e., forward regression), variables in the model may become nonsignificant after other variables enter the model, but are nevertheless retained because of the analytic approach. Sixth, it is also interesting to consider that oftentimes the independent variable(s) selected by the statistical criterion may not be physiologically justified.

Hierarchical regression requires the investigator to plan or justify the order of entry for each independent variable. Kerlinger (6) stated that, "the research problem and the theory behind the problem should determine the order of entry of variables in multiple regression analysis" (p. 545). Examples of hierarchical regression are the two nonexercise-based $\dot{V}o_2$ *max* prediction models by Malek and colleagues (13, 14). In both studies, the investigators initially entered traditional predictors such as age, height, and weight into the model and then entered habitual physical activity indices such as duration and intensity of their exercise. The goal of the investigators was to determine the unique contribution of habitual physical activity above and beyond the usual predictor variables used to predict $\dot{V}o_2$ *max*.

Research questions

The research questions that can be answered using multiple regression with continuous variables can be adopted for categorical variables. In addition, curvilinear regression may be used, for example, to develop prediction models for body composition equations using skinfold measurement (7, 8). More recently, curvilinear regression has been used in neuromuscular studies by Malek and Coburn (1–5, 9–12, 15) to describe the patterns of responses for electromyographic and mechanomyographic responses versus power (or torque) output during various exercise perturbations for the three superficial quadriceps muscles.

The output below uses curvilinear regression based on powered vectors to determine the patterns of responses for electromyographic amplitude during incremental cycle ergometry. It should be noted that the term "normalized" indicates that each subject's data were adjusted relative to their maximal value and then multiplied by 100. For example, if a subject achieved a maximal power output of 200 watts, and data were recorded at 80, 110, 140, 170, and 200 watts, then the normalized power output would be 40, 55, 70, 85, and 100 percent. Thereafter, the normalized output can either squared (x^2) or cubed (x^3) in order to develop the quadratic or cubic model, respectively.

Using SPSS pulldown menu for curvilinear (powered vectors) regression analysis

1. Click **Analyze,** then move cursor over Regression, and then move cursor over Linear and left click.
2. Click **EMG_amplitude_data_normalized** and move to Dependent box.
3. Click **Normalized_Power_Output** and move to Independent(s) box.
4. Click **Next.**
5. Click **Normalized_Power_Output_squared_X2** and move to Independent(s) box.
6. Click **Next.**
7. Click **Normalized_Power_Output_cubed_X3** and move to Independent(s) box.

   a. You should be on Block 3 of 3.

8. Click **OK.**

Syntax for SPSS curvilinear (powered vectors) regression analysis

REGRESSION
/MISSING LISTWISE
/STATISTICS COEFF OUTS R ANOVA CHANGE
/CRITERIA=PIN(.05) POUT(.10)

/NOORIGIN
/DEPENDENT EMG_amplitude_data_normalized
/METHOD=ENTER Normalized_Power_Output
/METHOD=ENTER Normalized_Power_Output_squared_X2
/METHOD=ENTER Normalized_Power_Output_cubed_X3.

Interpreting SPSS curvilinear (powered vectors) regression analysis

As shown in Table 9.2, this output indicates that each independent variable was entered (i.e., "Enter") into the model. Models 2 and 3 represent the quadratic and cubic models respectively.

As shown in Table 9.3, the Model Summary indicates whether or not the change in the R-square value is statistically significant. As shown in Model 3, the R-square change was not significantly (Sig. F. change = 0.087) different from Model 2. Therefore, in the present example, the quadratic model (Model 2) best-fit the relationship between normalized power output and normalized electromyographic amplitude.

As shown in Table 9.4, therefore using the values, from Model 2, in the "B" column, the powered vector model for this analysis would be: $Y = 0.241 + 0.001(x) + 0.736(x^2)$.

Table 9.2 Variables entered/removed, reprint courtesy of International Business Machines Corporation

Variables Entered/Removed[a]

Model	Variables entered	Variables removed	Method
1	Normalized_Power_Output		Enter
2	Normalized_Power_Output_squared_X2		Enter
3	Normalized_Power_Output_cubed_X3		Enter

Source: © International Business Machines Corporation.

Note
a Dependent Variable: EMG_amplitude_data_normalized.

Table 9.3 Model summary, reprint courtesy of International Business Machines Corporation

Model Summary

Model	R	R-square	Adjusted R-square	Std. error of the estimate	Change statistics				
					R-square change	F change	df1	df2	Sig. F change
1	.929[a]	.864	.862	.0933202555	.864	715.902	1	113	.000
2	.946[b]	.896	.894	.0819358494	.032	34.583	1	112	.000
3	.948[c]	.899	.896	.0812177136	.003	2.989	1	111	.087

Source: © International Business Machines Corporation.

Notes
a Predictors: (Constant), Normalized_Power_Output.
b Predictors: (Constant), Normalized_Power_Output, Normalized_Power_Output_squared_X2.
c Predictors: (Constant), Normalized_Power_Output, Normalized_Power_Output_squared_X2, Normalized_Power_Output_cubed_X3.

Table 9.4 Coefficients, reprint courtesy of International Business Machines Corporation

Coefficients[a]

Model		Unstandardized coefficients		Standardized coefficients	t	Sig.
		B	Std. error	Beta		
1	(Constant)	.028	.022		1.310	.193
	Normalized_Power_Output	.882	.033	.929	26.756	.000
2	(Constant)	.241	.041		5.900	.000
	Normalized_Power_Output	.001	.153	.001	.009	.993
	Normalized_Power_Output_squared_X2	.736	.125	.945	5.881	.000
3	(Constant)	.105	.088		1.191	.236
	Normalized_Power_Output	.923	.554	.972	1.666	.099
	Normalized_Power_Output_squared_X2	−1.009	1.017	−1.296	−.993	.323
	Normalized_Power_Output_cubed_X3	.974	.563	1.303	1.729	.087

Source: © International Business Machines Corporation.

Note

a Dependent Variable: EMG_amplitude_data_normalized.

Write-up for curvilinear (powered vectors) regression analysis

In the current study, curvilinear regression applying powered vectors was used to determine the relationship between normalized EMG amplitude versus power output. The results indicated that the best-fit model was quadratic ($R = 0.946$, $p < 0.001$) for the composite data.

Using SPSS pulldown menu for regression analysis with dummy coding

1. Click **Analyze,** then move cursor over Regression, and then move cursor over Linear and left click.
2. Click **Vo₂max_ml** and move to Dependent box.
3. To move the variables dummy coded for race:
   a. Click on "White."
   b. Hold down the Shift key.
   c. Click on "African_American."
   d. This will highlight the three dummy coded categories.
   e. Move them into Block 1.
4. Click **Next.**
5. Click **wt_kg** and move to Independent(s) box.
6. Click **ht_meter** and move to Independent(s) box.
7. Click **age_yrs** and move to Independent(s) box.
8. Click **Next.**
9. Click **timeperw** and move to Independent(s) box.
10. Click **intensity** and move to Independent(s) box.
    a. You should be on Block 3 of 3.

11. Click **Statistics**.

    a.   Make sure the R-squared change box is checked.

    b.   Click **Continue**.

12. Click **OK**.

Syntax for regression analysis with dummy coding

REGRESSION
/MISSING LISTWISE
/STATISTICS COEFF OUTS R ANOVA CHANGE
/CRITERIA=PIN(.05) POUT(.10)
/NOORIGIN
/DEPENDENT Vo_2mx_ml
/METHOD=ENTER White Latino African_American
/METHOD=ENTER wt_kg ht_meter age_yrs
/METHOD=ENTER timeperw intensity.

Interpreting regression analysis with dummy coding

As shown in Table 9.5, this indicates that each independent variable was entered into the model. That is, we first accounted for any potential variance accounted for by race (Model 1), and then accounted for other variables in Models 2 and 3.

As shown in Table 9.5, the Model Summary table indicates that race did not significantly contribute to the model ($p = 0.301$), whereas the variables in Models 2 ($p = 0.000$, as shown) and 3 ($p = 0.001$) significantly contributed to the regression model. Therefore, Model 3 is the model that best-fits the data.

As shown in Table 9.7, for Model 3, the variables that significantly contributed to the overall regression model are weight, height, age, and intensity of training variables. Therefore, the final regression equation would only use the coefficient values from these variables.

Write-up for curvilinear (powered vectors) regression analysis

The write-up would be similar to the sample write-up in Chapter 8.

Table 9.5 Variables entered/removed, reprint courtesy of International Business Machines Corporation

Variables Entered/Removed[a]

Model	Variables entered	Variables removed	Method
1	African_American, White, Latino[b]		Enter
2	age_yrs, wt_kg, ht_meter[b]		Enter
3	Times/wk_exercise, intensity of subjects training (6–20)[b]		Enter

Source: © International Business Machines Corporation.

Notes
a Dependent Variable: Vo_2mx_ml.
b All requested variables entered.

Table 9.6 Model summary, reprint courtesy of International Business Machines Corporation
Model Summary

Model	R	R-square	Adjusted R-square	Std. error of the estimate	Change statistics				
					R-square change	F change	df1	df2	Sig. F change
1	.223[a]	.050	.010	433.109	.050	1.243	3	71	.301
2	.689[b]	.475	.428	329.125	.425	18.317	3	68	.000
3	.758[c]	.575	.524	300.421	.101	7.808	2	66	.001

Source: © International Business Machines Corporation.

Notes
a Predictors: (Constant), African_American, White, Latino.
b Predictors: (Constant), African_American, White, Latino, age_yrs, wt_kg, ht_meter.
c Predictors: (Constant), African_American, White, Latino, age_yrs, wt_kg, ht_meter, Times/wk_exercise, intensity of subjects training (6–20).

Table 9.7 Coefficients, reprint courtesy of International Business Machines Corporation
Coefficients[a]

Model	Unstandardized coefficients		Standardized coefficients	t	Sig.
	B	Std. error	Beta		
1 (Constant)	−2405.516	1111.853		−2.164	.034
White	−66.016	127.572	−.064	−.517	.607
Latino	47.014	116.248	.051	.404	.687
African_American	118.638	114.887	.123	1.033	.306
wt_kg	17.441	5.836	.319	2.988	.004
ht-meter	1834.825	716.270	.283	2.562	.013
age_yrs	−11.715	3.997	−.257	−2.931	.005
Times/wk_exercise	11.597	15.683	.063	.739	.462
Intensity of subjects training (6–20)	90.637	25.023	.350	3.622	.001

Source: © International Business Machines Corporation.

Note
a Dependent Variable: Vo_2mx_ml.

Note

1. In some cases, prior to using powered vectors regression the data will need to be centered to provide a more logical interpretation of the y-intercept. We refer the reader to Pedhazur EJ (*Multiple regression in behavioral research*. Orlando, FL: Harcourt Brace, 1997).

References

1. Coburn JW, Housh TJ, Cramer JT, Weir JP, Miller JM, Beck TW, Malek MH, and Johnson GO. Mechanomyographic time and frequency domain responses of the vastus medialis muscle during submaximal to maximal isometric and isokinetic muscle actions. *Electromyography and Clinical Neurophysiology* 44: 247–255, 2004.

2. Coburn JW, Housh TJ, Cramer JT, Weir JP, Miller JM, Beck TW, Malek MH, and Johnson GO. Mechanomyographic and electromyographic responses of the vastus medialis muscle during isometric and concentric muscle actions. *Journal of Strength and Conditioning Research/National Strength & Conditioning Association* 19: 412–420, 2005.

3. Coburn JW, Housh TJ, Malek MH, Weir JP, Cramer JT, Beck TW, and Johnson GO. Mechanomyographic and electromyographic responses to eccentric muscle contractions. *Muscle & Nerve* 33: 664–671, 2006.

4. Coburn JW, Housh TJ, Malek MH, Weir JP, Cramer JT, Beck TW, and Johnson GO. Neuromuscular responses to three days of velocity-specific isokinetic training. *Journal of Strength and Conditioning Research/National Strength & Conditioning Association* 20: 892–898, 2006.

5. Coburn JW, Housh TJ, Weir JP, Malek MH, Cramer JT, Beck TW, and Johnson GO. Mechanomyographic responses of the vastus medialis to isometric and eccentric muscle actions. *Medicine and Science in Sports and Exercise* 36: 1916–1922, 2004.

6. Kerlinger FN. *Foundations of behavioral research*. New York: Holt, Rinehart and Winston, 1986.

7. Lohman TG. Skinfolds and body density and their relation to body fatness: a review. *Human Biology* 53: 181–225, 1981.

8. Lohman TG. *Advances in body composition assessment*. Champaign, I.L.: Human Kinetics, 1992.

9. Malek MH, Coburn JW, and Tedjasaputra V. Comparison of electromyographic response for the superficial quadriceps muscles: cycle vs. knee-extensor ergometry. *Muscle & Nerve* 39: 810–818, 2009.

10. Malek MH, Coburn JW, and Tedjasaputra V. Comparison of mechanomyographic amplitude and mean power frequency for the rectus femoris muscle: cycle vs. knee-extensor ergometry. *Journal of Neuroscience Methods* 181: 89–94, 2009.

11. Malek MH, Coburn JW, Weir JP, Beck TW, and Housh TJ. The effects of innervation zone on electromyographic amplitude and mean power frequency during incremental cycle ergometry. *Journal of Neuroscience Methods* 155: 126–133, 2006.

12. Malek MH, Coburn JW, York R, Ng J, and Rana SR. Comparison of MMG sensors during incremental cycle ergometry for the quadriceps femoris. *Muscle & Nerve*, in press.

13. Malek MH, Housh TJ, Berger DE, Coburn JW, and Beck TW. A new non-exercise based VO_2max prediction equation for aerobically trained females. *Medicine and Science in Sports Exercise* 36: 1804–1810, 2004.

14. Malek MH, Housh TJ, Berger DE, Coburn JW, and Beck TW. A new non-exercise-based VO_2max prediction equation for aerobically trained men. *Journal of Strength and Conditioning Research/National Strength & Conditioning Association* 19: 559–565, 2005.

15. Malek MH, Housh TJ, Coburn JW, Weir JP, Schmidt RJ, and Beck TW. The effects of interelectrode distance on electromyographic amplitude and mean power frequency during incremental cycle ergometry. *Journal of Neuroscience Methods* 151: 139–147, 2006.

16. Marelich WD. Trend analysis, in: *Encyclopedia of research design*. NJ Salkind, ed. Thousand Oaks, C.A.: SAGE Publications, 2010, pp. 1535–1537.

10 Regression model validation

Introduction

When developing a prediction model, it is important to then determine if the model is valid. The validation of a regression model is important because it allows the investigator to compare the accuracy of the regression equation for the population used to develop the model. Holiday et al. (2) has stated that the "central tenet of cross-validation is that the custodians of the model should not release a prediction equation to the user community without some assurance that it will do a good job" (p. 616).

Traditionally, investigators have used data-splitting in which the sample is "split" into a derivation and validation group. In this approach, initially introduced by Mosier (5) in 1951, the investigator randomly selects cases from the total data set and assigns each case into a derivation and validation group. From there, the derivation group is used to develop the prediction model, whereas the validation group is then used to determine the validity of the new equation. Cooil et al. (1) stated that, "sample-splitting is *not* an efficient approach to cross-validation ... it can lead to larger prediction errors in the validation stage ... and a larger probability of type II error in the significance testing of the model" (p. 272).

PRESS statistic

The *Predicted Residual Sum of Squares* (PRESS) statistic is an attractive alternative to model validation, because it uses the entire data set and, therefore, avoids the need to split the data (2). The PRESS approach is similar to the statistical jack-knife approach in that it uses N-1 cases from the sample used to derive the equation (2). Therefore, using the PRESS statistic the investigator can estimate an R-squared (R^2_{PRESS}) and standard error of estimate (SEE_{PRESS}) value. These values (R^2_{PRESS} and SEE_{PRESS}) can be compared with the R^2 and SEE values from the regression model to determine the validity of the model. For example, Malek and colleagues (4) used the PRESS statistic and reported similar R^2 (0.67) and SEE values (247 ml min^{-1}) when compared to the R^2_{PRESS} (0.63) and SEE_{PRESS} (259 ml min^{-1}), respectively. It should be noted, that PRESS values were not derived from the validation group, but from the original sample used to generate the regression model. Holiday et al. stated, "The PRESS statistic and associated residuals do not require the data to be split, [and] yield alternative unbiased estimates of R^2 and SEE" (p. 612). Therefore in the example above, Malek et al. (4) concluded that their new equation for predicting $\dot{V}o_2$ *max* had high generalizability for the population of aerobically trained women.

Indices of validation

When validating a new regression model or cross-validating an existing equation there are a number of indices which traditionally have been used in the exercise science literature. The constant error (CE) is an index which examines the difference between the predicted and observed value. This value can be calculated for each subject.

$$CE = Observed_{value} - Predicted_{value} \qquad\qquad \textbf{(Equation 1)}$$

Another index is the total error (TE, equation 2) which is the best single criterion for determining the accuracy of an equation. As shown below, the TE combines the errors associated with the SEE (standard error of the estimate) and CE (3). Unfortunately, this function cannot be performed in SPSS, but can be calculated in Excel with the appropriate column values and calculation functions indicated in the formula.

$$TE = \sqrt{\sum (observed_{value} - predicted_{value})^2 / n} \qquad\qquad \textbf{(Equation 2)}$$

The Bland-Altman plot is a visual approach used to determine the agreement between two different variables (i.e., observed $\dot{V}O_2$ *max* and predicted $\dot{V}O_2$ *max*). Typically, a scatter plot is used to shown the scores with a *line of identity* from the origin which indicates agreement of the scores. Therefore, the more centralized the scores around the origin, the stronger the agreement between the scores. The Bland-Altman plot also allows the investigator to examine the spread (or variability) of the scores. This is achieved by examining the 95 percent limits of agreement which is ± 2 standard deviations. Therefore, if the majority of scores are outside this range, then the two measures have poor agreement and cannot be used in place of the other.

Research questions

The research question that can be answered is whether a newly developed prediction model or an existing model is valid. In the latter case, when validating an existing equation this is called *cross-validation*.

Sample write-up

There is no specific format to write the results of this section. Typically, you would report the PRESS statistic after you have reported the results of the regression analysis. For example, you may use the following phrase to describe the result of the PRESS statistic, "*In order to validate our regression model, we performed the PRESS statistic. The results indicated that the $R^2_{PRESS} = 0.51$ which was close to the R^2 value from the model ($R^2 = 0.53$).*"

References

1. Cooil B, Winer RS, and Rados DL. Cross-validation for prediction. *Journal of Marketing Research* 24: 271–279, 1987.

2. Holiday DB, Ballard JE, and McKeown BC. PRESS-related statistics: regression tools for cross-validation and case diagnostics. *Medicine and Science in Sports and Exercise* 27: 612–620, 1995.

3. Lohman TG. *Advances in body composition assessment.* Champaign, I.L.: Human Kinetics, 1992.

4. Malek MH, Housh TJ, Berger DE, Coburn JW, and Beck TW. A new non-exercise based Vo$_2$max prediction equation for aerobically trained females. *Medicine and Science in Sports and Exercise* 36: 1804–1810, 2004.

5. Mosier CI. Problems and designs of cross-validation. *Educational and Psychological Measurement* 11, 5–11, 1951.

11 Logistic regression

Introduction

Logistic regression is similar to the previously discussed regression analyses such that it is used to predict an outcome. The one major difference between the typical ordinary least squares (OLS) regression model and logistic regression is that the dependent variable in the latter is binary or multinomial (i.e., categorical). That is, the outcome variable is discrete such as yes or no, or in a multinomial example, multiple categories (for example, types of "attack players" in volleyball; see Marcelino et al. [2]). Logistic regression can provide the probability or odds of an event occurring or not occurring. For example, it may be used to predict whether various factors will increase the risk of having a stroke. In this case, the outcome variable, stroke, is binary – either yes it will occur or no it will not occur. Alternatively, logistic regression could be used to determine what factors contribute to whether or not students in a clinical program such as physical therapy will pass or fail their state licensing board examination, or tactical factors contributing to success of attack players in volleyball. Essentially, application of logistic regression is similar to OLS regression, but with a categorical outcome.[1]

Besides categorical outcomes, how else does logistic regression differ from standard OLS regression? In OLS regression, significance of the overall regression model is assessed using F at the $p < 0.05$ or better level, testing to see if there is a significant amount of variability in the outcome variable accounted for by the linear combination of predictor variables (significance indicates the model R^2 exceeds an $R^2_{pop} = 0$). Logistic regression takes a slightly different approach due to the nature of the categorical outcome utilizing a maximum-likelihood approach. Applying maximum-likelihood, the predictors and outcome (binary or multinomial) are used to derive a set of predicted data-points which are then compared to the observed data-points. Significance of the overall logistic regression model is assessed using χ^2 at the $p < 0.05$ or better level, testing to see if "fit" of the predicted data to the observed data is superior to a model with no predictors (known as a null hypothesis model). A significant χ^2 indicates the hypothesized model is superior to the null hypothesis model.

As stated earlier, logistic regression can be applied just like OLS regression. Various outcomes can be modeled using individual predictors, or a set of predictors. Hierarchical models that are researcher driven can be designed, as can exploratory statistical models (e.g., stepwise). Individual predictors can be evaluated for their contribution and importance in hypothesized models. In addition, logistic regression can be used to predict group membership – in such applications models are built to enhance classification results.

Research questions

As discussed in the introduction section, the types of research questions answered by using logistic regression are those that have a dichotomous outcome (i.e., yes/ no), or are multinomial (three or more categories). The independent variables, however, do not need to be dichotomous. For example, we may use predictors such as resting heart rate, maximal heart rate, total blood cholesterol, and stress level to predict whether or not a person will have a heart attack or not. As in OLS regression, however, categorical predictors with three or more levels need to be specially coded (e.g., dummy coded, effect coded) prior to use.

There are a number of statistical assumptions associated with logistic regression which are similar to OLS regression. As with all of the tests covered in this textbook, many of these assumptions will be familiar to you, and thus not assessed here. They include an adequate sample size, linearity of the predictors and the logit-transformed outcome (but avoid multicollinearity of the predictors), and absence outliers in each level of the outcome variable for the predictors.

In the example below, the researcher is predicting whether or not subjects can be categorized into having severe or moderate muscle weakness in the quadriceps femoris muscles by using predictors such as time in physical therapy since they were diagnosed for muscle weakness, and whether or not they are currently diabetic. We purposefully kept this example simple to provide a clear and concise approach of presenting the statistical output. That is, with additional predictor variables (categorical and/or continuous) the output can become more complex to interpret especially in cases where the researcher is new to using this logistic regression.

Using SPSS pulldown menu for logistic regression

1. Click **Analysis**, then move cursor over Regression, and then move cursor over Binary Logistic and left click.
2. Click **level_of_muscle_weakness** and move to Dependent box.
3. Click **time_in_physical_therapy** and move to Block 1 of 1.
4. Click **diabetic** and move to Block 1 of 1.
5. *Note: The "Categorical" does not need to be used in this example, however, when a predictor variable has three or more categories such as exercise intensity (low, moderate, and high) then the "Categorical" button can be used.*
6. Click **Save**.

   a. Check box for Probabilities.
   b. Check box for Group membership.
   c. Click **Continue**.

7. Click **Options**.

   a. Check box for Classification plots.
   b. Check box for Hosmer-Lemeshow goodness-of-fit (*an additional model-fit test*).

    c. Note: The researcher can change the Probability for Stepwise values which are defaulted to Entry = 0.05 Removal = 0.10 in cases which are justified. Also the Maximum Iterations values is set at a default value of 20, but that can also be changed by the researcher in cases which are justified.

    d. Click **Continue**.

8.   Click **OK**.

Syntax for SPSS for logistic regression

```
LOGISTIC REGRESSION VARIABLES Muscle_Weakness
/METHOD=ENTER Time_in_physical_therapy Diabetic
/SAVE=PRED PGROUP
/CLASSPLOT
/PRINT=GOODFIT
/CRITERIA=PIN(0.05) POUT(0.10) ITERATE(20) CUT(0.5).
```

Interpreting the output for logistic regression

As shown in Tables 11.1 and 11.2, respectively, SPSS will initially provide information regarding how many cases will be used as well as information about the dependent variable. In this example, therefore, we have 80 cases with no missing data, and the dependent variable is categorical (40 with severe muscle weakness, and 40 with moderate muscle weakness).

Table 11.1 Case processing summary, reprint courtesy of International Business Machines Corporation

Case Processing Summary

Unweighted cases[a]		N	Percent
Selected cases	Included in analysis	80	100.0
	Missing cases	0	.0
	Total	80	100.0
Unselected cases		0	.0
Total		80	100.0

Source: © International Business Machines Corporation.

Note
a If weight is in effect, see classification table for the total number of cases.

Table 11.2 Dependent variable encoding, reprint courtesy of International Business Machines Corporation

Dependent Variable Encoding

Original value	Internal value
severe	0
moderate	1

Source: © International Business Machines Corporation.

Table 11.3 (Block 0) provides information about the model in which there are no predictor values and, therefore, would be akin to the null hypothesis (where no predictors significantly contributed to the criterion variable). Nevertheless, the table indicates what would be the predictive power of the model if all subjects were in the default group (i.e., moderate muscle weakness). In this example, the overall predictive capacity of the model is 50 percent. This makes sense since half of our study subjects are severe in muscle weakness, while the other half are moderate – the technique with no predictors in the model merely places everyone into the moderate category, yielding the 50 percent success rate.

Table 11.4 (Block 1) provides information about the model containing the two predictors. The Omnibus Tests of Model Coefficients is akin to the overall significant test seen in the regression chapter. Therefore, the significant values indicate that the two predictors are contributing to the model. Table 11.5 (Model Summary) provides information regarding the predictive capacity of this model. The "–2 Log likelihood" is akin to a chi-square, whereas the two R-square values (referred to as *pseudo R^2's*) are similar to the R-square values in multiple regression with the caveat that the values in Table 11.3 are calculated using maximum-likelihood least squares instead of the ordinary least squares which is typically used in multiple regression. Nevertheless, most researchers will report the "Nagelkerke R-square" rather than the "Cox & Snell R-Square" value, because the former is based on a scale ranging from 0 to 1.0, whereas

Table 11.3 Block 0: beginning block, reprint courtesy of International Business Machines Corporation

Block 0: Beginning Block
Classification Table[a,b]

Observed			Predicted level of muscle weakness		Percentage correct
			Severe	*Moderate*	
Step 0	Level of muscle weakness	Severe	0	40	.0
		Moderate	0	40	100.0
	Overall percentage				50.0

Source: © International Business Machines Corporation.

Notes
a Constant is included in the model.
b The cut value is .500.

Table 11.4 Block 1: method=enter, reprint courtesy of International Business Machines Corporation

Block 1: Method=Enter
Omnibus Tests of Model Coefficients

		Chi-square	*df*	*Sig.*
Step 1	Step	81.385	2	.000
	Block	81.385	2	.000
	Model	81.385	2	.000

Source: © International Business Machines Corporation.

the latter has a maximum value of 0.75 (in the present example, the "Nagelkerke R-square" is greater than the "Cox & Snell R-Square" value).

The "Hosmer and Lemeshow Test" which is shown in Table 11.6 is not significant ($p > 0.05$), which is a good thing as we want this type of model test to be nonsignificant. The finding of this test indicates the observed rate of events matches the expected rate of events. Thus, a nonsignificant finding indicates the observed and expected rate of events are similar. The "Contingency Table for Hosmer and Lemeshow Test" (Table 11.7) provides information similar to the crosstabs. The table applies the resulting muscle weakness grouping strategy (based on the model) into nine percentiles, which allows for comparisons of the observed and expected cell frequencies for fit. For example, Step 4 for the severe muscle weakness group shows an observed cell frequency of 8 and an

Table 11.5 Model summary, reprint courtesy of International Business Machines Corporation

Model Summary

Step	−2 Log likelihood	Cox & Snell R-square	Nagelkerke R-square
1	29.519[a]	.638	.851

Source: © International Business Machines Corporation.

Note
a Estimation terminated at iteration number 6 because parameter estimates changed by less than .001.

Table 11.6 Hosmer and Lemeshow test, reprint courtesy of International Business Machines Corporation

Hosmer and Lemeshow Test

Step	Chi-square	df	Sig.
1	12.552	7	.084

Source: © International Business Machines Corporation.

Table 11.7 Contingency table for Hosmer and Lemeshow test, reprint courtesy of International Business Machines Corporation

Contingency Table for Hosmer and Lemeshow Test

		Level of muscle weakness = severe		Level of muscle weakness = moderate		Total
		Observed	Expected	Observed	Expected	
Step 1	1	11	10.869	0	.131	11
	2	8	7.816	0	.184	8
	3	8	7.675	0	.325	8
	4	8	7.616	0	.384	8
	5	3	3.934	4	3.066	7
	6	1	1.393	10	9.607	11
	7	0	.472	8	7.528	8
	8	0	.142	6	5.858	6
	9	1	.083	12	12.917	13

Source: © International Business Machines Corporation.

expected cell frequency of 7.616. Both are similar suggesting good fit. Looking across the table, all of the observed and expected cell frequencies are very similar (see Hosmer and Lemeshow [1], for additional information on table interpretation).

The "Classification Table" (Table 11.8) shows great improvement over the null hypothesis model. Table 11.8 shows 38 subjects predicted to have severe muscle weakness, whereas 40 subjects were predicted to have moderate muscle weakness. The "Percentage correct" column indicates that the prediction for the two categories is high (95 and 100 percent, respectively). Moreover, the overall predictive capacity of the model is 97.5 percent which is greater than the 50 percent value for the overall predictive capacity shown in Table 11.3.

The "Variables in the Equation" (Table 11.9) is similar to the "Coefficients" table when performing OLS regression. That is, of the two predictors (time in physical therapy and currently diabetic) only the time in physical therapy significantly contributed to the model as a predictor. The predictor of whether or not the subject is currently diabetic did not significantly contribute to the model ($p = 0.883$). When interpreting the column labeled "Exp(B)" in the table, for every unit of increase physical therapy time, the odds of being in the moderate muscle weakness category increases 1.965 times. This shows the benefits of physical therapy in terms of reducing pain. That is, the longer one is in physical therapy the more likely they will be in the moderate muscle weakness category. Since being a diabetic isn't a significant predictor, the odds are not interpreted.

Table 11.8 Classification table, reprint courtesy of International Business Machines Corporation

Classification Table[a]

Observed			Predicted level of muscle weakness		Percentage correct
			Severe	*Moderate*	
Step 1	Level of muscle weakness	**Severe**	38	0	95.0
		Moderate	0	40	100.0
	Overall percentage				97.5

Source: © International Business Machines Corporation.

Note
a The cut value is .500.

Table 11.9 Variables in the equation, reprint courtesy of International Business Machines Corporation

Variables in the Equation

		B	S.E.	Wald	df	Sig.	Exp(B)
Step 1[a]	Time in physical therapy	.676	.140	23.305	1	.000	1.965
	currently diabetic (yes/no)	.175	1.187	.022	1	.883	1.191
	Constant	−5.190	1.352	14.731	1	.000	.006

Source: © International Business Machines Corporation.

Note
a Variable(s) entered on step 1: time in physical therapy, currently diabetic (yes/no).

Although the overall model is good based on the chi-square test of the model coefficients and the Hosmer and Lemeshow test, only time in physical therapy is a solid predictor. If our research interest was to broadly model muscle weakness categories, then the significance of the individual predictors isn't as important as the overall model findings. However, in most instances, researchers report both the overall model findings and individual predictor results.

Sample write-up for logistic regression

Logistic regression was performed using two groups of subjects as the outcome; 40 individuals having severe muscle weakness in the quadriceps femoris muscles, and 40 individuals having moderate muscle weakness. Two variables were investigated as predictors of muscle weakness category: time in physical therapy since they were diagnosed for muscle weakness, and whether or not they are currently diabetic. A logistic regression model with the two predictors was significant, χ^2 (2, N=80)=81.385, $p<0.05$, with a Nagelkerke pseudo R^2 of 0.85. The Hosmer and Lemeshow test also showed the model to be acceptable, χ^2 (7, N=80)=12.552, $p=0.084$. Model classification results were good, with 97.5 percent of the cases correctly classified per their observed categories. Looking at the individual regression coefficients, according to the Wald criterion, only time in physical therapy was significant, χ^2 (1, N=80)=23.305, $p<0.05$. The odds ratio for this predictor shows that for every unit of increase in physical therapy time, individuals are 1.965 times more likely to be in the moderate muscle weakness group than the severe muscle weakness group. Overall, the model with two predictors did well to predict those with severe and moderate muscle weakness. These findings also underscore the importance of time in physical therapy, that is, with longer periods leading to a greater likelihood of being in the moderate muscle weakness group instead of severe weakness group.

Example 2 (hierarchical logistic regression)

In this second example, the researcher extends the aim of the above example by inserting another predictor variable. Specifically, the researcher is interested in knowing whether or not the patient's habitual exercise history is a predictor for determining their muscle weakness. The predictor variable, therefore, is the number of 30-minute walks the patient performs on a weekly basis during the last 2 years. Moreover, the researcher is interested in knowing if accounting for this variable would influence the contribution of the other two predictors: time in physical therapy and whether or not the patient is diabetic. Thus, the researcher will need to perform a hierarchical logistic regression.

Using SPSS pulldown menu for logistic regression (example 2)

1. Click **Analysis**, then move cursor over Regression, and then move cursor over Binary Logistic and left click.
2. Click **level_of_muscle_weakness** and move to Dependent box.
3. Click **number_of_30_min_walks_weekly** and move to Block 1 of 1.
4. Click Next.

    a.   Click **time_in_physical_therapy** and move to Block 2 of 2.
    b.   Click **diabetic** and move to Block 2 of 2.

5. Click **Save**.

    a. Check box for Probabilities.
    b. Check box for Group membership.
    c. Click **Continue**.

6. Click **Options**.

    a. Check box for Classification plots.
    b. Check box for Hosmer-Lemeshow goodness-of-fit (*an additional model-fit test*).
    c. Note: The researcher can change the Probability for Stepwise values which are defaulted to Entry = 0.05 Removal = 0.10 in cases which are justified. Also the Maximum Iterations value is set at a default value of 20, but that can also be changed by the researcher in cases which are justified.
    d. Click **Continue**.

7. Click **OK**.

Syntax for SPSS for logistic regression (example 2)

```
LOGISTIC REGRESSION VARIABLES Muscle_Weakness
/METHOD=ENTER number_of_30_min_walks_weekly
/METHOD=ENTER Time_in_physical_therapy Diabetic
/SAVE=PRED PGROUP
/CLASSPLOT
/PRINT=GOODFIT
/CRITERIA=PIN(0.05) POUT(0.10) ITERATE(20) CUT(0.5).
```

Interpreting the output for hierarchical logistic regression

Tables 11.10 and 11.11, respectively, are identical to Tables 11.1 and 11.2 and, therefore, provide the same relevant information.

Table 11.12 (Block 0) again provides the same information about Table 11.3. That is, in a model with no predictors the overall predictive capacity of the model is 50 percent.

Table 11.10 Case processing summary, reprint courtesy of International Business Machines Corporation

Case Processing Summary

Unweighted cases[a]		N	Percent
Selected cases	Included in analysis	80	100.0
	Missing cases	0	.0
	Total	80	100.0
Unselected cases		0	.0
Total		80	100.0

Source: © International Business Machines Corporation.

Note
a If weight is in effect, see classification table for the total number of cases.

Table 11.11 Dependent variable encoding, reprint courtesy of International Business Machines Corporation

Dependent Variable Encoding

Original value	Internal value
severe	0
moderate	1

Source: © International Business Machines Corporation.

Table 11.12 Block 0: beginning block, reprint courtesy of International Business Machines Corporation

Block 0: Beginning Block
Classification Table[a,b]

	Observed		Predicted level of muscle weakness		Percentage correct
			Severe	Moderate	
Step 0	Level of muscle weakness	Severe	0	40	.0
		Moderate	0	40	100.0
	Overall percentage				50.0

Source: © International Business Machines Corporation.

Notes
a Constant is included in the model.
b The cut value is .500.

Table 11.13 (Block 1) provide information about the model containing the single predictor (habitual exercise activity). As noted earlier, the Omnibus Test of Model Coefficients is an overall significance test. Thus, the significant values indicated that the single predictor is contributing to the model. Table 11.14 (Model Summary) provides information regarding the predictive capacity of this model. The "Nagelkerke R-square" rather than the "Cox & Snell R-Square" value is the pseudo R-square value to be evaluated because the former is based on a scale ranging from 0 to 1.0, whereas the latter has a maximum value of 0.74.

The "Hosmer and Lemeshow Test" (Table 11.15) indicates a nonsignificant finding ($p = 0.831$). This indicates the observed rate of events matches the expected rate of events. The "Contingency Table for Hosmer and Lemeshow Test" (Table 11.16) shows that the observed cell frequencies (for either the severe or moderate muscle weakness groups) compare well to the expected cell frequencies.

The "Classification Table" (Table 11.17) shows a great improvement over the null hypothesis model. Table 11.17 shows 31 subjects predicted to have severe muscle weakness, whereas 37 subjects were predicted to have moderate muscle weakness. The "Percentage correct" column indicates that the prediction for the two categories is high (77.5 and 92.5 percent, respectively). In addition, the overall predictive capacity of the model is 85.0 percent which is greater than the 50 percent value for the overall predictive capacity shown in Table 11.12.

Table 11.13 Block 1: method = enter, reprint courtesy of International Business Machines Corporation

Block 1: Method = Enter
Omnibus Tests of Model Coefficients

		Chi-square	df	Sig.
Step 1	Step	64.953	1	.000
	Block	64.953	1	.000
	Model	64.953	1	.000

Source: © International Business Machines Corporation.

Table 11.14 Model summary, reprint courtesy of International Business Machines Corporation
Model Summary

Step	−2 Log likelihood	Cox & Snell R-square	Nagelkerke R-square
1	45.950[a]	.556	.741

Source: © International Business Machines Corporation.

Note
a Estimation terminated at iteration number 7 because parameter estimates changed by less than .001.

Table 11.15 Hosmer and Lemeshow test, reprint courtesy of International Business Machines Corporation

Hosmer and Lemeshow Test

Step	Chi-square	df	Sig.
1	1.478	4	.831

Source: © International Business Machines Corporation.

Table 11.16 Contingency table for Hosmer and Lemeshow test, reprint courtesy of International Business Machines Corporation
Contingency Table for Hosmer and Lemeshow Test

		Level of muscle weakness = severe		Level of muscle weakness = moderate		Total
		Observed	Expected	Observed	Expected	
Step 1	1	12	11.904	0	.096	12
	2	19	19.833	3	2.167	22
	3	9	7.659	10	11.341	19
	4	0	.570	12	11.430	12
	5	0	.033	9	8.967	9
	6	0	.002	6	5.998	6

Source: © International Business Machines Corporation.

The "Variables in the Equation" (Table 11.18) indicates that the habitual exercise activity predictor did significantly contribute to the model. Moreover, interpreting the odds labeled "Exp(B)" in the table, for every unit of increased habitual exercise activity, the odds of being in the moderate muscle weakness category increases 13.549 times.

We next add the original two predictors from Example 1 as a block into the model to evaluate their effects after accounting for habitual exercise activity. As shown in Figure 11.1, for Block 2, the overall model is significant, χ^2 (3, N = 80) = 92.785, with a strong Nagelkerke R-square. Thus, a model with all three variables is tenable. Because the model is hierarchical, we can also directly evaluate whether the two added variables significantly contribute to the overall model with habitual exercise activity already in the model. The line labeled "Block" shows χ^2 (2, N = 80) = 27.831, $p < 0.001$; above and beyond the initial model with habitual exercise activity, the addition of time in physical therapy and diabetic diagnosis as a block significantly contribute to the model.

We can now return to the overall model findings. Figure 11.2 shows the "Hosmer and Lemeshow Test," the "Contingency Table for Hosmer and Lemeshow Test," and the "Classification Table." The Hosmer and Lemeshow Test shows a nonsignificant finding ($p = 0.547$) indicating the observed rate of events matches the expected rate of events. A review of the contingency table indicates good fit between the observed and expected cell frequencies. The "Classification Table" indicates that the

Table 11.17 Classification table, reprint courtesy of International Business Machines Corporation

Classification Table[a]

Observed			Predicted level of muscle weakness		Percentage correct
			Severe	Moderate	
Step 1	Level of muscle weakness	Severe	31	9	77.5
		Moderate	3	37	92.5
	Overall percentage				85.0

Source: © International Business Machines Corporation.

Note
a The cut value is .500.

Table 11.18 Variables in the equation, reprint courtesy of International Business Machines Corporation

Variables in the Equation

		B	S.E.	Wald	df	Sig.	Exp(B)
Step 1[a]	Number_of_30_min_walks_weekly	2.606	.609	18.327	1	.000	13.549
	Constant	−4.820	1.150	17.562	1	.000	.008

Source: © International Business Machines Corporation.

Note
a Variable(s) entered on step 1: number_of_30_min_walks_weekly.

Block 2: Method = Enter

Omnibus Tests of Model Coefficients

		Chi-square	df	Sig.
Step 1	Step	27.831	2	.000
	Block	27.831	2	.000
	Model	92.785	2	.000

Model Summary

Step	−2 Log likelihood	Cox & Snell R Square	Nagelkerke R Square
1	18.119[a]	.686	.915

a. Estimation terminated at iteration number 8 because parameter estimates changed by less than .001.

Figure 11.1 Block 2: method = enter, reprint courtesy of International Business Machines Corporation.

Source: © International Business Machines Corporation.

predictive capacity of the model is 97.5 percent which is greater than the 50 percent value for Block 0 and the 85 percent value for Block 1.

As shown in Table 11.19, of the three predictors in the model, habitual exercise activity ($p = 0.023$), time in physical therapy ($p = 0.001$), and currently diabetic ($p = 0.318$), the first two significantly contribute to the model. Importantly, a closer examination of the "Exp(B)" column indicates that for every one unit of increase in habitual exercise activity, the odds of being in the moderate muscle weakness category increases to 14.734, and for every one unit of increase in physical therapy time, the odds of being in the moderate muscle weakness category increases 1.785 times. As with our first example, this second example again shows the benefits of physical therapy in terms of reducing pain. That is, the longer one is in physical therapy the more likely they will be in the moderate muscle weakness category. Moreover, having a greater impact is habitual exercise activity. That is, those with a history of walking regularly are more likely to experience moderate muscle weakness.

Table 11.19 Variables in the equation, reprint courtesy of International Business Machines Corporation

Variables in the Equation

		B	S.E.	Wald	df	Sig.	Exp(B)
Step 1[a]	Number_of_30_min_walks_weekly	2.690	1.183	5.171	1	.023	14.734
	Time in physical therapy	.579	.180	10.400	1	.001	1.785
	Currently diabetic (no/yes)	1.471	1.472	.999	1	.318	4.352
	Constant	−9.842	3.257	9.134	1	.003	.000

Source: © International Business Machines Corporation.

Note
a Variable(s) entered on step 1: time in physical therapy, currently diabetic (no/yes).

Hosmer and Lemeshow Test

Step	Chi-square	df	Sig.
1	6.906	8	.547

Contingency Table for Hosmer and Lemeshow Test

		Level of muscle weakness = severe		Level of muscle weakness = moderate		Total
		Observed	Expected	Observed	Expected	
Step 1	1	8	7.998	0	.002	8
	2	7	6.991	0	.009	7
	3	9	8.954	0	.046	9
	4	8	8.730	0	.270	9
	5	6	6.127	2	1.873	8
	6	0	1.028	8	6.972	8
	7	1	.141	7	7.859	8
	8	0	.029	8	7.971	8
	9	0	.002	8	7.998	8
	10	0	.000	7	7.000	7

Classification Table[a]

			Predicted		
			Level of muscle weakness		Percentage Correct
	Observed		Severe	Moderate	
Step 1	Level of muscle weakness	Severe	39	1	97.5
		Moderate	1	39	97.5
	Overall Percentage				97.5

a. The cut value is .500

Figure 11.2 Hosmer and Lemeshow test, reprint courtesy of International Business Machines Corporation.

Source: © International Business Machines Corporation.

Sample write-up for logistic regression (example 2)

Hierarchical logistic regression was performed using two groups of subjects as the outcome; 40 individuals having severe muscle weakness in the quadriceps femoris muscles, and 40 individuals having moderate muscle weakness. Three variables were investigated as predictors of muscle weakness category: habitual exercise history operationalized as the number of 30-minute walks per week, time in physical therapy since they were diagnosed for muscle weakness, and whether or not they are currently diabetic. Hierarchical logistic regression was performed, first evaluating habitual exercise history as a single predictor of muscle weakness category, then evaluating time in physical therapy and diabetic diagnosis as predictors. The first model with habitual exercise activity was significant, χ^2 (1, N = 80) = 64.953,

$p < 0.001$, with a Nagelkerke pseudo R^2 of 0.741. The Hosmer and Lemeshow test also showed the model to be acceptable, χ^2 (4, N = 80) = 1.478, $p = 0.831$. Model classification results were good, with 85 percent of the cases correctly classified per their observed categories. Looking at the individual regression coefficients, according to the Wald criterion, habitual exercise history (i.e., 30-minute walks per week) was significant, χ^2 (1, N = 80) = 18.327, $p < 0.001$. The odds ratio for this predictor shows that for every unit of increase in 30-minute walks per week, individuals are 13.549 times more likely to be in the moderate muscle weakness group than the severe muscle weakness group.

A second set of predictors was next added to the model; time in physical therapy and whether or not they are currently diabetic. These two variables as a block added significantly to the earlier model with habitual exercise activity as the sole predictor, χ^2 (2, N = 80) = 27.831, $p < 0.001$. With all three variables included, the overall model was good, χ^2 (3, N = 80) = 92.785, $p < 0.001$, supported by the Hosmer and Lemeshow test, χ^2 (8, N = 80) = 6.906, $p = 0.547$, and a Nagelkerke R Square value of 0.915. Model classification results improved, with 97.5 percent of the cases correctly classified per their observed categories. Looking at the individual regression coefficients, according to the Wald criterion, habitual exercise history (i.e., 30-minute walks per week) remained significant, χ^2 (1, N = 80) = 5.171, $p = 0.023$. The odds ratio for this predictor shows that for every unit of increase in 30-minute walks per week, individuals are 14.734 times more likely to be in the moderate muscle weakness group than the severe muscle weakness group. In addition, time in physical therapy was significant, χ^2 (1, N = 80) = 10.40, $p = 0.001$. The odds ratio for this predictor shows that for every unit of increase in physical therapy time, individuals are 1.785 times more likely to be in the moderate muscle weakness group than the severe muscle weakness group. Overall, the model with all three predictors did well to predict those with severe and moderate muscle weakness. In particular, higher levels of habitual exercise activity and time in physical therapy led to a greater likelihood of being in the moderate muscle weakness group instead of the severe weakness group.

Note

1. We often get asked by students and colleagues why one can't use binary outcomes in OLS regression since such variables are often used as predictors. In the circumstance of a binary outcome in OLS regression, the resulting predicted values will often exceed the maximum outcome value of 1, an impossible value!

References

1. Hosmer DW and Lemeshow S. *Applied logistic regression*. New York: Wiley, 2000.
2. Marcelino R, Afonso J, Moraes JC, and Mesquita I. Determinants of attack players in high-level men's volleyball. *Kinesiology* 46: 234–241, 2014.

Part III
Special statistical procedures

12 Multivariate analysis of variance (MANOVA)

Introduction

MANOVA is a statistical procedure to determine mean differences between independent groups for more than one dependent variable that is continuous. MANOVA, in part, may be viewed as an extension of ANOVA, where only one continuous dependent variable is examined. Although MANOVA is not typically used in studies examining physiological outcomes, it may be an effective statistical tool in the case where multiple dependent variables should be analyzed together. For example, the National Football League (NFL) has their annual Combine where elite collegiate football players undergo multiple functional tests to determine various outcome measures such as speed, agility, power, and strength, Moreover, these players are categorized into the positions they play (i.e., linebacker, offensive line, running back, etc.). Thus, one potential application of MANOVA may be to determine whether or not the results of these functional tests are influenced by the position the athlete plays.

Separate ANOVAs could be run using each of these outcome measures separately (e.g., separate analyses for speed, agility, power, and strength). However, because these outcomes correlate with each other, the findings might be misleading. If group differences were found on each of these outcomes, it's possible the resulting differences are due to the "shared variance" across the outcomes due to their correlations. The advantage of MANOVA is that the overlapping variance is accounted for, leading to a more appropriate assessment of group differences.

Although MANOVA is the appropriate choice over ANOVA when dependent variables are correlated, the technique is laden with statistical assumptions from both ANOVA and OLS regression. In addition, MANOVA is less robust to assumption violations, and can be less sensitive to revealing group differences than standard univariate techniques if dependent variables are not correlated.

Research questions

As noted above, the types of research questions answered by MANOVA are similar to those for ANOVA, except that instead of one outcome or dependent variable, there are multiple dependent variables that form a multivariate composite. This composite is formed by linearly combining the dependent variables in such a way as to maximize group differences. The standard research question asks: Do groups differ on the multivariate composite of outcome variables?

To this end, a single multivariate test statistic is derived and assessed for significance. Follow-up tests for significant multivariate findings are then performed using Roy-Bargmann stepdown tests, which are used to discover the dependent variable(s) that evidence group differences, adjusting for their variance overlap. Group differences on the dependent variables are assessed by entering the dependent variables one-at-a-time into the model (i.e., hierarchical entry), with each dependent variable acting as a covariate for subsequent dependent variables entered into the model.

There are a number of statistical assumptions associated with MANOVA similar to ANOVA. For example, equality of cell sizes, normality, and homogeneity of variance are all assessed in the typical manner (see Chapter 4). In addition, multivariate normality and homogeneity of variance are also assessed. There are also assumptions related to multiple regression (covered in Chapter 7) assessed due to the multiple dependent variables in the model, including linearity and absence of multicollinearity and singularity. The dependent variables are required to be correlated as well – if the outcomes show no correlation, ANOVAs on the dependent variables separately are the appropriate approach.

In the example below, strength and speed are used as dependent variables, whereas group is the independent variable. These two variables correlate at −0.758. The group variable has two levels (wide receivers and offensive linemen). Therefore, in this example, we are performing a one-way MANOVA[1] with strength and speed as the dependent variables.

Using SPSS pulldown menu for one-way MANOVA (example 1)

1. Click **Analyze,** then move the cursor over **Multivariate** then left click.
2. Click **Group,** then move it to the Fixed Factor(s) box.
3. *Holding the CTRL key down,* click **Strength and Speed** and move them to the Dependent Variables box.
4. Click **Descriptives** (*in newer versions of SPSS click the Options box*).

    a. Check the boxes for Descriptive statistics and Homogeneity tests.
    b. Click **Group,** then move to Display Means for box (*Note: In the newer version of SPSS, you will need to click the EM Means button to perform the option below*).

        i. Then click Compare Main Effects.

            1. Under Confidence Interval Adjustment select LSD from the pulldown menu.

    c. Then click **Continue.**

5. Click **Plots.**

    a. Then click **Group** and move to Horizontal Axis.
    b. Click **Add.**
    c. Click **Continue.**

6. Click **OK.**

Syntax for SPSS for one-way MANOVA (example 1)

GLM Strength Speed BY Group
/METHOD=SSTYPE(3)
/INTERCEPT=INCLUDE
/PLOT=PROFILE(Group) TYPE=LINE ERRORBAR=NO MEANREFERENCE=NO
YAXIS=AUTO
/EMMEANS=TABLES(Group) COMPARE ADJ(LSD)
/PRINT=DESCRIPTIVE HOMOGENEITY
/CRITERIA=ALPHA(.05)
/DESIGN= Group.

Note: The "/Plot" statement may not work in older SPSS versions as this is the syntax generated with SPSS version 25. Please refer to ANOVA sections for how to plot data set.

Interpreting the output for one-way MANOVA (example 1)

As shown in Table 12.1, IBM SPSS Statistics software (SPSS) generates the Between-Subjects Factors table. This table provides information regarding the two groups we are examining. The next table (Table 12.2) is the Descriptives Statistics table which provides the means, standard deviations, and N for the two dependent variables (strength and speed) for each of the two groups (wide receivers and offensive linemen).

Table 12.1 Between-subjects factors, reprint courtesy of International Business Machines Corporation

Between-Subjects Factors

		Value label	*N*
Positions	0	Wide_receivers	40
	1	Offensive_linemen	39

Source: © International Business Machines Corporation.

Table 12.2 Descriptive statistics, reprint courtesy of International Business Machines Corporation

Descriptive Statistics

	Positions	*Mean*	*Std. deviation*	*N*
Strength Index	Wide_receivers	64.8250	5.75521	40
	Offensive_linemen	84.7179	8.47271	39
	Total	74.6456	12.31742	79
Speed Index	Wide_receivers	84.1000	6.68255	40
	Offensive_linemen	49.7179	6.08254	39
	Total	67.1266	18.42891	79

Source: © International Business Machines Corporation.

Table 12.3 presents the results for the Box's Test of Equality of Covariance Matrices. Essentially, this test indicates whether or not the observed covariance matrices of the outcome (dependent) variables are equal across the three groups, serving as an assessment of multivariate homogeneity of variance. As shown in Table 12.3, the p-value, in this example, is $p = 0.110$ and is therefore not statistically significant. It should be noted, however, that instead of using a p-value of 0.05 as the demarcation, a very stringent p-value of 0.001 is used to determine whether or not this test is statistically significant.

Table 12.4 shows the Multivariate Tests which allows us to determine whether or not there is a significant effect for group on all the outcome variables. This is, in part, akin to determining whether or not the overall F-ratio is statistically significant in a one-way ANOVA. Thus, as shown in Table 12.4, Pillai's Trace is revealed to be statistically significant ($p < 0.001$).[2]

As shown in Table 12.5, the Tests of Between-Subjects Effects is essentially the univariate tests for the effects of group on each of the outcome variables. Thus, this is akin to having two one-way ANOVAs with no adjustments for the correlated

Table 12.3 Box's test of equality of covariance matrices, reprint courtesy of International Business Machines Corporation

Box's Test of Equality of Covariance Matrices[a]

Box's M	6.207
F	2.011
df1	3
df2	1090273.816
Sig.	.110

Source: © International Business Machines Corporation.

Notes
Tests the null hypothesis that the observed covariance matrices of the dependent variables are equal across groups.
a Design: Intercept + Group.

Table 12.4 Multivariate tests, reprint courtesy of International Business Machines Corporation

Multivariate Tests[a]

Effect		*Value*	*F*	*Hypothesis df*	*Error df*	*Sig.*
Intercept	Pillai's Trace	.995	8243.177[b]	2.000	76.000	.000
	Wilks' Lambda	.005	8243.177[b]	2.000	76.000	.000
	Hotelling's Trace	216.926	8243.177[b]	2.000	76.000	.000
	Roy's Largest Root	216.926	8243.177[b]	2.000	76.000	.000
Group	Pillai's Trace	.905	362.939[b]	2.000	76.000	.000
	Wilks' Lambda	.095	362.939[b]	2.000	76.000	.000
	Hotelling's Trace	9.551	362.939[b]	2.000	76.000	.000
	Roy's Largest Root	9.551	362.939[b]	2.000	76.000	.000

Source: © International Business Machines Corporation.

Notes
a Design: Intercept + Group.
b Exact statistic.

Table 12.5 Tests of between-subjects effects, reprint courtesy of International Business Machines Corporation

Tests of Between-Subjects Effects

Source	Dependent variable	Type III sum of squares	df.	Mean square	F	Sig.
Corrected Model	Strength Index	7814.404[a]	1	7814.404	149.691	.000
	Speed Index	23343.237[b]	1	23343.237	571.066	.000
Intercept	Strength Index	441600.328	1	441600.328	8459.203	.000
	Speed Index	353611.389	1	353611.389	8650.707	.000
Group	Strength Index	7814.404	1	7814.404	149.691	.000
	Speed Index	23343.237	1	23343.237	571.066	.000
Error	Strength Index	4019.672	77	52.204		
	Speed Index	3147.497	77	40.877		
Total	Strength Index	452019.000	79			
	Speed Index	382463.000	79			
Corrected Total	Strength Index	11834.076	78			
	Speed Index	26490.734	78			

Source: © International Business Machines Corporation.

Notes
a R Squared = .660 (Adjusted R Squared = .656).
b R Squared = .881 (Adjusted R Squared = .880).

dependent variables. Nevertheless, for all outcome variables the overall *F*-ratio were significant (all *p*-values <0.001). In a typical ANOVA, the next step is to perform the follow-up test to determine which group means are statistically different from one another for each of the outcome variables. As shown in Figure 12.1, the Univariate Test is the one-way ANOVA and indicates that the overall *F*-ratio for strength and speed is statistically significant. Since we only have two groups, a post-hoc test is not needed, but for illustration purposes we have provided the Pairwise Comparisons table along with the Estimated Marginal Means table (Figure 12.1). Because the LSD (Least Significant Difference) was used for mean comparisons (no adjustment for increased Type I error), this should be assessed at the 0.01 level instead of 0.05. Regardless, there were significant mean differences between groups for strength and speed, respectively.

Although it may seem obvious that groups differ on both dependent variables, due to the high correlation (−0.758) between the variables, a proper assessment adjusting for this overlap is warranted. The technique used in this instance is the Roy-Bargmann stepdown test, which utilizes an alternative syntax approach in SPSS (see below). These stepdown tests are analogous to performing ANCOVAs using one of the dependent variables as a covariate. With three or more dependent variables, dependent variables are layered in one by one, evaluating the effects of each dependent variable with effects of the others accounted for. The order for layering dependent variables into the stepdown analyses is determined by the researcher based on study hypotheses. Whichever order is decided by the investigator, as in ANCOVA applications, the homogeneity of regression assumption should be assessed prior to performing the Roy-Bargmann test since adjustments are being made to the dependent variables by the other variables in the model.

Estimated Marginal Means
Positions

Estimates

Dependent Variable	Positions	Mean	Std. Error	95% Confidence Interval	
				Lower Bound	Upper Bound
Strength Index	Wide_receivers	64.825	1.142	62.550	67.100
	Offensive_linemen	84.718	1.157	82.414	87.022
Speed Index	Wide_receivers	84.100	1.011	82.087	86.113
	Offensive_linemen	49.718	1.024	47.679	51.757

Pairwise Comparisons

Dependent Variable	(I) Positions	(J) Positions	Mean Difference (I-J)	Std. Error	Sig.[b]	95% Confidence Interval for Difference[b]	
						Lower Bound	Upper Bound
Strength Index	Wide_receivers	Offensive_linemen	−19.893*	1.626	.000	−23.131	−16.655
	Offensive_linemen	Wide_receivers	19.893*	1.626	.000	16.655	23.131
Speed Index	Wide_receivers	Offensive_linemen	34.382*	1.439	.000	31.517	37.247
	Offensive_linemen	Wide_receivers	−34.382*	1.439	.000	−37.247	−31.517

Based on estimated marginal means

*. The mean difference is significant at the .05 level.

b. Adjustment for multiple comparisons: Least Significant Difference (equivalent to no adjustments)

Univariate Tests

Dependent Variable		Sum of squares	df	Mean Square	F	Sig.
Strength Index	Contrast	7814.404	1	7814.404	149.691	.000
	Error	4019.672	77	52.204		
Speed Index	Contrast	23343.237	1	23343.237	571.066	.000
	Error	3147.497	77	40.877		

The F tests the effect of Positions. This test is based on the linearly independent pairwise comparisons among the estimated marginal means.

Figure 12.1 Estimated marginal means, reprint courtesy of International Business Machines Corporation.

Source: © International Business Machines Corporation.

In our current example using strength and speed as dependent variables, for the Roy-Bargmann test, we will first evaluate group differences on speed, followed by strength. Therefore, in the Roy-Bargmann tests, speed will be evaluated first, and then used as a covariate to evaluate strength. A quick check using syntax from the ANCOVA chapter on homogeneity of regression shows no violation of the assumption ($p > 0.05$). The special MANOVA syntax from SPSS is used for the Roy-Bargmann tests, specifying "stepdown" in the print command. Thus, you will first need to open a new syntax page in order to type the following commands and perform the analyses. To open a new syntax file perform the following steps:

1. Move the cursor to **File** and then click.
2. Go to **New**, and then move to the cursor to **Syntax**.
3. Click on **Syntax** and a new file will open.
4. After the syntax has been written (see below), highlight the entire syntax and then press the green ▶ button near the top of the syntax window.
5. There will be several tables presented in the output display.

   a. Go to the table labeled Roy-Bargmann Stepdown F – tests (see below).

MANOVA
SPEED STRENGTH BY GROUP (0,1)
/PRINT = SIGNIF (**STEPDOWN**), ERROR (COR)
/METHOD UNIQUE
/DESIGN.

Roy-Bargmann stepdown F – tests (example 1)

Variable	Hypoth. MS	Error MS	StepDown F	Hypoth. DF	Error DF	Sig. of F
Speed	23343.23674	40.87659	571.06615	1	77	.000
Strength	1018.86987	52.85908	19.27521	1	76	.000

Results of the stepdown tests first show differences between wide receivers and offensive linemen in terms of speed as the solitary dependent variable. After accounting for speed in the model, strength differences are still evident in offensive linemen.

Sample write-up for one-way MANOVA (example 1)

A one-way MANOVA was performed to determine differences in football positions on two functional tests: speed and strength. Box's Test of Equality of Covariance Matrices was not significant ($p = 0.110$), meeting the assumption of multivariate homogeneity of variance. The MANOVA revealed significant [Pillai's Trace = 0.91, $F(2, 76) = 362.939$, $p < 0.001$] group effects for the multivariate composite of strength and speed. Roy-Bargmann stepdown tests are next performed to evaluate group differences on the dependent variables, with the higher-priority dependent variable being speed. Results show groups differed on speed, $F_{stepdown}(1, 77) = 571.07$, $p < 0.001$. Using observed mean values, wide receivers are faster than offensive linemen ($M = 84.1$ vs. $M = 49.7$). After accounting for speed, strength also yielded significant group differences, $F_{stepdown}(1, 76) = 19.28$, $p < 0.001$, with offensive linemen being stronger than wide receivers (observed $M = 84.7$ vs. $M = 64.8$). As might be expected, wide receivers are faster, while offensive linemen are stronger.

Factorial MANOVA (example 2)

Here, we have added another factor with two levels to the previous example. Therefore, we still have group (wide receivers and offensive linemen), but now have added whether or not they played at a Division I academic institution. The dependent variables are still strength and speed indices. Thus, in this example, we are performing a factorial MANOVA with strength and speed as the outcomes variables.

Using SPSS pulldown menu for factorial MANOVA (example 2)

1. Click **Analyze**, then move the cursor over **Multivariate** then left click.
2. Click **Group**, then move it to the Fixed Factor(s) box.
3. Click **College_Division**, then move it to the Fixed Factor(s) box.
4. *Holding the CTRL key down*, click **Strength and Speed** and move them to the Dependent Variables box.

5. Click **Descriptives** (*in newer versions of SPSS click the Options box*).

   a. Check the boxes for Descriptive statistics and Homogeneity tests.
   b. *Holding down the CTRL key*, and click **Group, College_Division, and Group*College_Division**, then move to Display Means for box (*Note: In the newer version of SPSS, you will need to click the EM Means button to perform the option below*).

      i. Then click Compare Main Effects.

         1. Under Confidence Interval Adjustment select LSD from the pull-down menu.

   c. Then click **Continue.**

6. Click **Plots.**

   a. Then click **Group** and move to Horizontal Axis.
   b. Then click **College_Division** and move to Separate Lines.
   c. Click **Add.**
   d. Click **Continue.**

7. Click **Paste.**

   a. The syntax below will appear in a new syntax window.
   b. For the line starting with /EMMEANS=TABLES(Group*College_Division) modify the syntax to:

      i. /EMMEANS=TABLES(Group*College_Division) Compare(College_Division).

8. Then highlight the entire syntax and press the green ▶ at the top of the syntax.

Syntax for SPSS for factorial MANOVA (example 2)

```
GLM Strength Speed BY Group College_Division
/METHOD=SSTYPE(3)
/INTERCEPT=INCLUDE
/PLOT=PROFILE(Group*College_Division)      TYPE=LINE      ERRORBAR=NO
MEANREFERENCE=NO YAXIS=AUTO
/EMMEANS=TABLES(Group) COMPARE ADJ(LSD)
/EMMEANS=TABLES(College_Division) COMPARE ADJ(LSD)
/EMMEANS=TABLES(Group*College_Division) Compare(College_Division)
/PRINT=DESCRIPTIVE HOMOGENEITY
/CRITERIA=ALPHA(.05)
/DESIGN= Group College_Division Group*College_Division.
```


Interpreting the output for factorial MANOVA (example 2)

As shown in Table 12.6, SPSS generates the Between-Subjects Factors table similar to Table 12.1. In this table, however, college division is the second factor and whether or not the subjects are from Division 1 academic institutions.

Table 12.6 Between-subjects factors, reprint courtesy of International Business Machines Corporation

Between-Subjects Factors

		Value label	*N*
Positions	0	Wide_receivers	40
	1	Offensive_linemen	39
College division	0	NCAA D1	43
	1	Non-NCAA D1	39

Source: © International Business Machines Corporation.

Table 12.7 presents the results for the Box's Test of Equality of Covariance Matrices for this factorial MANOVA example. Similar to example 1, the test is not statistically significant ($p = 0.947$) and, thus, using a p-value of 0.001 as the cutoff for the level of statistical significance it can be concluded that the assumption was met.

Table 12.8 shows the Multivariate Tests which allows us to determine whether or not there is a significant effect for group, college division, and/or the group × college division interaction term. In this example, Pillai's Trace is statistically significant for each factor (group and college division) as well as for the interaction term.

As shown in Table 12.9, the Tests of Between-Subjects Effects provides information regarding the effect of group, college division, and the interaction term (group × college division) on each of the outcome variables (strength and speed). In this example, the interaction term is statistically significant for both the strength ($p = 0.018$) and speed ($p = 0.017$) index. The focus of the follow-up testing should be on the group × college division interaction for the strength and speed indices. In this case, the follow-up test will focus on determining mean differences between positions across college divisions. As shown in Figure 12.2, the table for Univariate Tests indicates that there was no significant overall F-ratio for the strength index for the wide receiver position ($p = 0.072$), whereas for the offensive linemen position the overall F-ratio was significant ($p < 0.001$). Therefore, the table for Pairwise Comparisons indicates that for the strength index there was a significant mean difference

Table 12.7 Box's test of equality of covariance matrices, reprint courtesy of International Business Machines Corporation

Box's Test of Equality of Covariance Matrices[a]

Box's M	3.552
F	.365
df1	9
df2	54714.650
Sig.	.947

Source: © International Business Machines Corporation.

Notes
Tests the null hypothesis that the observed covariance matrices of the dependent variables are equal across groups.
a Design: Intercept + Group + College_Division + Group*College_Division.

Table 12.8 Multivariate tests, reprint courtesy of International Business Machines Corporation

Multivariate Tests[a]

Effect		Value	F	Hypothesis df	Error df	Sig.
Intercept	Pillai's Trace	.997	10594.226[b]	2.000	74.000	.000
	Wilks' Lambda	.003	10594.226[b]	2.000	74.000	.000
	Hotelling's Trace	286.330	10594.226[b]	2.000	74.000	.000
	Roy's Largest Root	286.330	10594.226[b]	2.000	74.000	.000
Group	Pillai's Trace	.914	390.761[b]	2.000	74.000	.000
	Wilks' Lambda	.086	390.761[b]	2.000	74.000	.000
	Hotelling's Trace	10.561	390.761[b]	2.000	74.000	.000
	Roy's Largest Root	10.561	390.761[b]	2.000	74.000	.000
College_Division	Pillai's Trace	.284	14.690[b]	2.000	74.000	.000
	Wilks' Lambda	.716	14.690[b]	2.000	74.000	.000
	Hotelling's Trace	.397	14.690[b]	2.000	74.000	.000
	Roy's Largest Root	.397	14.690[b]	2.000	74.000	.000
Group*College_Division	Pillai's Trace	.133	5.666[b]	2.000	74.000	.005
	Wilks' Lambda	.867	5.666[b]	2.000	74.000	.005
	Hotelling's Trace	.153	5.666[b]	2.000	74.000	.005
	Roy's Largest Root	.153	5.666[b]	2.000	74.000	.005

Source: © International Business Machines Corporation.

Notes

a Design: Intercept + Group + College_Division + Group*College_Division.

b Exact statistic.

Table 12.9 Tests of between-subjects effects, reprint courtesy of International Business Machines Corporation

Tests of Between-Subjects Effects

Source	Dependent variable	Type III sum of squares	df.	Mean square	F	Sig.
Corrected Model	Strength Index	8968.262[a]	3	2989.421	78.235	.000
	Speed Index	23729.755[b]	3	7909.918	214.867	.000
Intercept	Strength Index	432967.765	1	432967.765	11331.016	.000
	Speed Index	349570.814	1	349570.814	9495.840	.000
Group	Strength Index	7299.365	1	7299.365	191.029	.000
	Speed Index	22867.961	1	22867.921	621.192	.000
College_Division	Strength Index	947.565	1	947.565	24.798	.000
	Speed Index	159.160	1	159.160	4.323	.041
Group*College_Division	Strength Index	223.990	1	223.990	5.862	.018
	Speed Index	219.842	1	219.842	5.972	.017
Error	Strength Index	2865.814	75	38.211		
	Speed Index	2760.979	75	36.813		
Total	Strength Index	452019.000	79			
	Speed Index	382463.000	79			
Corrected Total	Strength Index	11834.076	78			
	Speed Index	26490.734	78			

Source: © International Business Machines Corporation.

Notes
a R Squared = .758 (Adjusted R Squared = .748).
b R Squared = .896 (Adjusted R Squared = .892).

Positions* College Division

Estimates

Dependent Variable	Positions	College Division	Mean	Std. Error	95% Confidence Interval	
					Lower Bound	Upper Bound
Strength Index	Wide_receivers	NCAA D1	66.524	1.349	63.837	69.211
		Non-NCAA D1	62.947	1.418	60.122	65.772
	Offensive_linemen	NCAA D1	89.227	1.318	86.602	91.853
		Non-NCAA D1	78.882	1.499	75.896	81.869
Speed Index	Wide_receivers	NCAA D1	87.048	1.324	84.410	89.685
		Non-NCAA D1	80.842	1.392	78.069	83.615
	Offensive_linemen	NCAA D1	49.500	1.294	46.923	52.077
		Non-NCAA D1	50.000	1.472	47.069	52.931

Pairwise Comparisons

Dependent Variable	Positions	(I) College Division	(J) College Division	Mean Difference (I-J)	Std. Error	Sig.[b]	95% Confidence Interval for Difference[b]	
							Lower Bound	Upper Bound
Strength Index	Wide_receivers	NCAA D1	Non-NCAA D1	3.576	1.957	.072	−.323	7.475
		Non-NCAA D1	NCAA D1	−3.576	1.957	.072	−7.475	.323
	Offensive_linemen	NCAA D1	Non-NCAA D1	10.345*	1.996	.000	6.368	14.321
		Non-NCAA D1	NCAA D1	−10.345*	1.996	.000	−14.321	−6.368
Speed Index	Wide_receivers	NCAA D1	Non-NCAA D1	6.206*	1.921	.002	2.379	10.032
		Non-NCAA D1	NCAA D1	−6.206*	1.921	.002	−10.032	−2.379
	Offensive_linemen	NCAA D1	Non-NCAA D1	−.500	1.959	.799	−4.403	3.403
		Non-NCAA D1	NCAA D1	.500	1.959	.799	−3.403	4.403

Based on estimated marginal means
*. The mean difference is significant at the .05 level.
b. Adjustment for multiple comparisons: Least Significant Difference (equivalent to no adjustments)

Univariate Tests

Dependent Variable	Positions		Sum of squares	df	Lower Bound	F	Sig.
Strength Index	Wide_receivers	Contrast	127.590	1	127.590	3.339	.072
		Error	2865.814	75	38.211		
	Offensive_linemen	Contrast	1026.269	1	1026.269	26.858	.000
		Error	2865.814	75	38.211		
Speed Index	Wide_receivers	Contrast	384.121	1	384.121	10.434	.002
		Error	2760.979	75	36.813		
	Offensive_linemen	Contrast	2.397	1	2.397	.065	.799
		Error	2760.979	75	36.813		

Each F tests the simple effects of College Division within each level combination of the other effects shown.
These tests are based on the linearly independent pairwise comparisons among the estimated marginal means.

Figure 12.2 Positions college division, reprint courtesy of International Business Machines Corporation.

Source: © International Business Machines Corporation.

between offensive linemen from Division 1 academic institutions (89.2 ± 1.3) compared to non-Division 1 academic institutions (78.9 ± 1.5). In a similar manner, for the speed index we find that the overall *F*-ratio is not significant for the offensive linemen ($p = 0.799$), but is significant for the wide receivers ($p = 0.002$). Therefore, wide receivers from Division 1 academic institutions (87.0 ± 1.3) were faster than wide receivers from non-Division 1 academic institutions (80.8 ± 1.4).

Given the significant multivariate tests, as performed in example 1, we next run Roy-Bargmann stepdown tests. Using strength and speed as the dependent variables, for the Roy-Bargmann test we type the following syntax:

MANOVA
SPEED STRENGTH BY GROUP (0,1) COLLEGE_DIVISION (0, 1)
/PRINT = SIGNIF (STEPDOWN), ERROR (COR)
/METHOD = UNIQUE
/DESIGN.

Roy-Bargmann stepdown F – tests for college division (example 2)

Variable	Hypoth. MS	Error MS	StepDown F	Hypoth. DF	Error DF	Sig. of F
Speed	159.16049	36.81305	4.32348	1	75	0.041
Strength	918.71860	38.69170	23.74459	1	74	0.000

Roy-Bargmann stepdown F – tests for group (example 2)

Variable	Hypoth. MS	Error MS	StepDown F	Hypoth. DF	Error DF	Sig. of F
Speed	22867.96112	36.81305	621.19171	1	75	0.000
Strength	702.81586	38.69170	18.16451	1	74	0.000

Roy-Bargmann stepdown F – tests group by college division (example 2)

Variable	Hypoth. MS	Error MS	StepDown F	Hypoth. DF	Error DF	Sig. of F
Speed	219.84159	36.81305	5.97184	1	75	0.017
Strength	194.98111	38.69170	5.03935	1	74	0.028

The Roy-Bargmann tests for the main effects continue to underscore group differences for both independent variables and are interpreted in the standard way, first evaluating Speed as the sole dependent variable, followed by Strength after adjusting for Speed in the model. Overall, both Speed and Strength differ for those in different college divisions, and for those who are wide receivers vs. linemen. For the significant interaction terms, we next perform simple effects, first with the speed index as the sole dependent variable, focusing on college division within group. That is, we are aiming to answer the following questions, "*Are there speed differences between college division wide receivers? How about for offensive linemen?*" This effectively follows the logic of the Roy-Bargmann stepdown tests, which focused first on Speed as the sole dependent variable. This is performed using the following syntax:

MANOVA SPEED BY GROUP (0,1) COLLEGE_DIVISION (0,1)
/METHOD = UNIQUE
/DESIGN GROUP, COLLEGE_DIVISION W GROUP (1), COLLEGE_DIVISION W GROUP (2).

Tests of significance for speed using UNIQUE sums of squares

Sources of variation	SS	DF	MS	F	Sig of F
WITHIN+RESIDUAL	2760.98	75	36.81		
GROUP	22867.96	1	22867.96	621.19	0.000
COLLEGE_DIVISION W GROUP(1)	384.12	1	384.12	10.43	0.002
COLLEGE_DIVISION W GROUP(2)	2.40	1	2.40	0.07	0.799
(Model)	23729.76	3	7909.92	214.87	0.000
(Total)	26490.73	78	339.62		

Again, following the logic of the Roy-Bargmann stepdown test, we next perform the simple effects test using speed as the covariate and strength as the dependent variable. That is, after accounting for speed in the model, we are asking the following questions, "*Are there strength differences between college division wide receivers? How about for offensive linemen?*" In order to achieve this analysis, the following syntax was used to generate the subsequent table.

MANOVA STRENGTH BY GROUP (0,1) COLLEGE_DIVISION (0,1) WITH SPEED
/METHOD = SEQUENTIAL
/DESIGN GROUP, COLLEGE_DIVISION W GROUP (1), COLLEGE_DIVISION W GROUP (2).

Tests of significance for strength using cov adj SEQUENTIAL sums of squares

Sources of variation	SS	DF	MS	F	Sig of F
WITHIN+RESIDUAL	2863.19	74	38.69		
REGRESSION	2.63	1	2.63	0.07	0.795
GROUP	740.72	1	740.72	19.14	0.000
COLLEGE_DIVISION W GROUP(1)	124.32	1	124.32	3.21	0.077
COLLEGE_DIVISION W GROUP(2)	1022.32	1	1022.32	26.42	0.000
(Model)	8970.89	4	2242.72	57.96	0.000
(Total)	11834.08	78	151.72		

Sample write-up for factorial MANOVA (example 2)

A factorial MANOVA was performed to determine differences in football positions and where or not players were from Division 1 academic institutions on two functional tests: speed and strength. The Box's Test of Equality of Covariance Matrices was not significant ($p = 0.947$), therefore, it was concluded that the assumption of multivariate homogeneity of variance was met. The MANOVA revealed significant main effects for group [Pillai's Trace = 0.91, $F(2,74) = 390.76$, $p < 0.001$] and college division [Pillai's Trace = 0.28, $F(2,74) = 14.69$, $p < 0.001$] for the multivariate composite of strength and speed. The MANOVA revealed significant [Pillai's Trace = 0.13, $F(2,74) = 5.67$, $p < 0.001$] group × college division for the multivariate composite of strength and speed. Roy-Bargmann stepdown tests are next performed to evaluate group differences on the dependent variables, with the higher-priority dependent variable being speed. The results for the main effect for college division revealed a significant finding for both Speed [$F_{stepdown}(1,75)=4.32$; $p=0.041$] and Strength [$F_{stepdown}(1,74)=23.74$; $p<0.001$]. Similarly, the results for the main effect for group revealed a significant finding for both Speed [$F_{stepdown}(1,75)=621.19$; $p<0.001$] and Strength [$F_{stepdown}(1,74)=18.16$; $p<0.001$]. The results for the inter-action effects revealed a significant finding for Speed, [$F_{stepdown}(1,75)=5.97$; $p=0.017$]. After accounting for speed, strength also yielded significant group differ-ences, [$F_{stepdown}(1,74)=5.04$; $p=0.028$]. Simple main effects testing is next initiated to further investigate the interaction findings. Using Speed as the sole dependent variable, simple main effects testing shows speed differences for wide receivers in Division I vs. non-Division 1, [$F(1,75)=10.43$; $p<0.01$], but not for offensive linemen, [$F(1,75)=0.07$; $p>0.05$]. Next, after accounting for Speed in the model as a covariate, simple main effects testing shows no significant strength differences at the 0.05 or better level for wide receivers in Division I vs. Division 2, [$F(1,74)=3.21$; $p=0.077$], but did evidence differences between offensive linemen in Division I vs. Division 2, [$F(1,74)=6.42$; $p<0.001$].

Notes

1. With only two levels of the independent variable, a MANOVA is technically a Hotelling's T^2, although many just refer to it as a MANOVA.
2. Because of its robustness to assumption violations, we recommend the use of Pillai's Trace as the test statistic of choice for MANOVA over Wilk's Λ (1, 2).

References

1. Olson CL. On choosing a test statistic in multivariate analysis of variance. *Psychological Bulletin* 83, 579–586, 1976.
2. Olson CL. Practical considerations in choosing a MANOVA test statistic: a rejoinder to Stevens. *Psychological Bulletin* 86: 1350–1352, 1979.

Index

Page numbers in **bold** denote tables, those in *italics* denote figures.